THE WIND
AT MY BACK

To my mother Julie, without whom I would not be alive today.

Thank you, Mum. I love you so much.

THE
WIND
AT MY
BACK

A memoir of cancer, love and endurance

JOSH
KOMEN

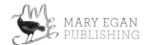

MARY EGAN
PUBLISHING

Published by Mary Egan Publishing
www.maryegan.co.nz

This edition published 2019

Designed, typeset and produced by Mary Egan Publishing
Cover designed by Anna Egan-Reid
Printed in China

ISBN 978-0-473-46429-5

CONTENTS

Foreword

To a scientist, acute leukaemia is a fascinating puzzle, a disease that is endlessly complicated, and which must be understood and rationally tackled. But to the patient, acute leukaemia is much more than that: it's frightening, confusing and, whatever the outcome, it's life-changing and for all too many life-ending. Leukaemia cells are smart. They have acquired the capacity for numerous alterations that increase their ability to multiply and survive and to replace healthy cells. Scientists may have invented exciting and groundbreaking treatments to suppress and destroy leukaemia, but the treating team knows that these treatments do not always work and even if they do, they unavoidably will injure, sometimes beyond repair, the person with leukaemia. In the detached vocabulary of the health service, treatment of acute leukaemia is an 'area of unmet need'.

On one ordinary day seven years ago, with no warning and for no reason at all, a completely ordinary young man fell right into that unholy mess. He'd grown up the same as anyone else, finished school and got out into the workforce. He had his family and lots of mates, loved his sports (and as a matter of fact was very successful at them). In short, he had the same happy expectations as any other 20-something-year-old with his whole life ahead of him. Imagine having to explain the problem to him. Much worse, imagine being the person who was having the problem explained. Josh Komen had been running to compete and win for his province, with a dream of running for New Zealand. Now he was going to have to run for himself.

This isn't a story about a new life-saving cure with an experimental treatment that succeeded when no one thought it could, when every other treatment had failed, the sort of story that gets written up in a scientific journal. It's about undergoing the available treatment, getting the leukaemia controlled and launching out in a new direction, only to be told that the leukaemia had come back. It's about undergoing further treatment (cruelly called 'salvage treatment', aiming to save what remains), being pushed down for weeks and becoming so ill that a month of life vanished while being unconscious in intensive care. It's about the gift of life, offered by an anonymous person from overseas, in the form of a bone marrow transplant. It's about enduring years of complications from that treatment and eventually being sent overseas to manage those complications.

But most of all it's about how an ordinary young man became extraordinary.

Because Josh has not been a passive recipient of all these strokes of fate. He has stood up after being bashed down. He has sucked it up. And he's pulled many others up along the way. I became ill during all of this. Josh always wanted to know how I was going before he would tell anything of himself. Directly or indirectly, lots of people with many different skills have been involved in Josh's care and he has become a friend of all he has met. For most of his time in Christchurch, years if it is all added up, he has lived at Ranui House and supported many other patients and families who have shared parts of his journey. He did the same when in Melbourne, Australia, for much of 2016, 2017 and 2018.

Far too many people have found themselves in Josh's shoes. More will be there this year, and every year to come. Josh is a compelling and fluent young man who is telling us about every one of these extraordinary people. His story reminds us again that we are not a product of what life throws at us, but rather that our lives can only be defined by what we do with what we have got.

Dr Peter Ganly
Medical Haematologist, BM, BCh, MA, PhD, FRACP, FRCPA

Introduction

As a mother, I find this hard to write. It brings back horrific memories of the times our family and Josh have endured. Tears roll down my cheeks. I have heard the words no mother should ever hear: 'Mum, please kill me. Mum, I want to die.'

A mother's job is to care, provide, to do the utmost to protect her children from pain and torment. All I could do was hold my son's hand and pray that he would live, find peace and happiness, and lead the life he was living before cancer.

Josh was strong, fit and happy before leukaemia. He was different to the other boys. After a night on the beers, he would be up at 7.30 am, running 25 km out on the Coast Road. He supplied his family with firewood, worked all the overtime he could and saved his money because he had dreams and ambitions. His determination set him apart from many of the people around him.

Then one day, cancer came into our lives uninvited. We were unprepared.

There were warning signs. You will read about the day he did the Lake Brunner bike race. He collapsed off his bike, sat outside the Moana petrol station drinking a Coke and eating a chocolate bar, willing himself to finish the ride.

I was waiting at the finish line. Other competitors approached me and said, 'Josh didn't look good.' I am amazed at how Josh got back on that bike and finished, pushing his way to Greymouth. His determination is a reflection of why he is still with us today. I will never forget the day we heard of Josh's diagnosis. We didn't know at the time that it was just the start of a journey the whole family would take. Dr Sharp called from Greymouth Hospital. He said, 'Please come here. I need to speak with you.' Walking in, I saw the look on the nurses' faces, and thought, *Something's not right with my boy.*

When we were told the news, my brother's arms flew up in the air and he said, 'I shouldn't be here!' but Dr Sharp said, 'You're family. You're all part of this now.'

He was right. The whole family was involved. My other two children stepped up to the mark to help and I was so proud of them both.

Josh went to the Christchurch Hospital Bone Marrow Unit. Leaving him there, I felt I had let him down, abandoned him to face this disease alone in his small isolation room. This situation was not in the parenting manual.

Every time I asked how he was, he'd say, 'I'll be okay, Mum.'

'Josh, will you really?' I'd ask.

He never let me know the full picture of his prognosis. I thought he was trying to shelter me from the reality of the situation, but I also wondered if keeping information from me was one of the few things he could still control, because the leukaemia was out of control.

I was angry, frustrated and scared. I wanted to know what was going on, but Josh was clever. I asked his doctor, Peter Ganly, what was going to happen. He said, 'Josh will tell you in his own time.' I knew Josh had gotten to him first!

I love my three wonderful children, four if you count my husband. My son Jacob was only 15 and Rachael was studying to be a teacher. They all needed a mother's comfort, but I had to help Josh. It felt selfish, but he needed me, and I needed to be there. I spent a lot of time walking in Christchurch's Hagley Park. I shed many tears there. If trees could talk, what stories they would tell.

I saw things a mother should never see. The screams of my son have haunted me for years. I held his hand when he was in a coma on life support and we didn't know if he would wake up. I held his hand through the transplant and the pain the GVHD (graft-versus-host disease) brought upon him, and I was there when he broke up with the girl he loved so dearly. The worst was the torture of trigeminal neuralgia. Josh screamed his heart out, wanting to die, when it felt like someone was stabbing his face. It nearly broke me. The look of fear on his face still haunts me today. I held my son's hand even though I was depleted, at my wits' end.

And there was more. Josh was in Australia when he had multiple heart attacks, over and over, calling me on the phone, telling me how much pain he was in. And yet his ultimate response was always, 'It'll be okay, Mum.'

'No Josh, please don't tell me this. You're not okay and I'm not there.'

I bought a ticket and flew to him, holding his hand through the relentless heart attacks while the doctors discussed what to do. It had always been Josh's dream to win gold for New Zealand and here we were in the Royal Melbourne Cardiac Unit. The Olympics were on TV and two of Josh's former competitors were running the 1500 metres.

The doctors came in and said, 'Well Josh, you've won the Gold Medal for the most discussed patient in the cardiac unit.'

It was never straightforward with Josh, never. All I could give my son was my hand and my love.

As a mother, you want to have all the answers for your children. The words, 'It'll be all right,' just didn't cut it because in Josh I saw anger, fear, frustration and sadness. You take it in, absorb it, swallow it, and put on the brave mother face because this is what you do. You suck it up and hold your child's hand because sometimes there are no words to express how much you want it all to go away.

For Josh, every day brings new challenges. Some days are good, others bad. I am proud of my family. Josh's pain has united us in a bond of love we could never have imagined. We talk, laugh, tease each other, and share a deep love. We know how tough life can be.

To any mother who faces challenges with their children, and feels helpless: hold their hand tight, rub their back, hold them close, and tell them you love them.

This is what I did. It's all I knew to do. I often ask Josh what I can do for him and his usual response is, 'Can you get me a new body?' I laugh and hug him. A mother can only do so much.

But I would, if only I could.

Julie Komen

The purpose through pain

When the pain and tiredness come, I am stuck in mud, in quicksand. It's a battle. I fight my own body. My head droops, my eyes ache, like the wrap of barbed wire at every blink. My neck bends under the weight of ten bricks. My face is burning, my eyes are like pinholes, fighting the fatigue. It's too much.

This is my daily life, the constant battle against my own body. I find it too hard to accept; in fact, I don't know who the person is who lives in this body. I keep screaming in my head, *What's happened to me? What the fuck is all this about? I'm too young to be an old man. I'm fucking 80 years old!* I'm 25 and have become an old man sitting in a rest home. I struggle to walk. Was I really one of the fastest 800-metre runners in New Zealand? Will I ever run again? Questions spin around in my head and scare the shit out of me. Is this life? Will the tiredness ever end? I have no answers.

A friend asks, 'Are you okay?' In my mind, I rage, *Of course I'm fucking not. I've been through all this shit and I can barely hold my body together!* I politely reply, 'Yeah bro, sweet. I'm just resting my eyes.'

I struggle to sit with my friends and engage with them, have a conversation. It's so hard to be with someone when you're in chronic pain and exhausted. I'm in another world, one where I don't want anyone else to be. I'm not myself. Will they still be my friend?

I can't quiet my inner voice. It starts screaming again: *I hate this. I hate my life. Why the fuck am I an old man at such a young age? Fucking cancer! Fucking chemo! Fuck everything.* Then I think, *Josh, breathe, just breathe. You've come this far. God is with you. You can fight this. Rest now. Wake up tomorrow and take one step forward. Accept that this is you now. Slow your mind down. All of this pain has a purpose and it won't be forever.*

The darkness falls and I sink into the bottomless hole of fatigue.

Will tomorrow be a better day?

PART ONE
GROWING UP

Success is not final,
failure is not fatal:
it is the courage to continue
that counts.

— WINSTON CHURCHILL

GREYMOUTH is a tough town. It can rain for weeks.

It's a rare, unique rain, seen only here. Harsh, cold, dripping right through to your bones, relentless, punishing. It can be frustrating and depressing. People sigh, 'More rain ...' But then the rain goes and the sun shines in a majestic heaven. The deep green of the bush opens your eyes wide. It's beautiful and you think, 'Wow! Do I really live here?'

From my home, I hear the crash of the ocean and the hum of cicadas in the hills. The sky is so blue, the gentle sea breeze is like a silky-soft blanket. To me, Greymouth is heaven on earth.

I think the West Coast of New Zealand reflects the way life is. Stormy and harsh, with days of relentless rain, just like tough days where we say, 'Stuff this. What am I doing living here? What am I doing at all?' Then the sun shines and we forget about the dismal, cold rainy days. Life is good. Nothing is a problem. We swim, surf, have BBQs, laugh and play. The Coast is a playground for the adventurous, so pure, so physical. I loved growing up here. I thrived in the sunshine and embraced running in the rain. It was cleansing and healing.

Greymouth is a hard-working coal mining and timber town. Tough, generous, respectful people with good, well-established values and a community backbone of volunteering, particularly in sport, coaching, mentoring and helping out after work and on the weekend. It's a community where everyone knows each other. If you misbehaved, Mum and Dad would always find out. This was my town, hard but fair, challenging at times, but rewarding. Every day of my Greymouth childhood was worth its weight in gold. My home town instilled in me the value that life is not easy, but if you work, and work hard enough – keep pushing through those cold, rainy days – the sun will shine again and you'll forget about the grey, bitter times.

Because this is life: never constant, always changing, good and bad, up and down. Appreciating the good and embracing the challenges. Appreciating other people, and life itself. This was my town. Greymouth.

Barefoot freedom

I was born the colour purple on June 10th 1987, then hurried away by nurses to the incubator room where I was watched carefully for several hours. It was a dramatic start, and not the only time I would be carted off with my life on the line.

My parents Julie and Peter were distraught. They didn't know where I was. Mum had endured all the pain and suffering of labour and her gift, her prize, had been whisked away. Mum and Dad didn't see or hold me for hours. They were so afraid I might not come back to them.

Apparently Mum had been given an injection and I had inadvertently received the whole dose. Mum was traumatised when she found out, white as a ghost, full of questions and wanting nothing more than to hold her new baby. It was a shaky start for us all.

I have a close and loving family: Mum, Dad, me, my sister Rachael and brother Jacob. My cousins Nick, Ben, Jon, Rhys, Matt, Tyler and Hannah are like brothers and sisters too, our closeness established through my beautiful Nanna Jean, the rock of our family.

Nanna was a determined, kind lady who worked as a nurse until she was 82. She looked after just about every member of the Greymouth community at one time or another, and her care went outside of the hospital. A jar of blackberry jelly or chocolate chip biscuits were likely at any time to appear in your letterbox. I often went with Nanna and my cousins to the Nelson Creek swimming hole or out to Punakaiki with a packed lunch and a cricket set, to swim, eat and play.

Swimming in the lagoon every day, climbing trees, doing what we liked: the world was ours. We were carefree. The occasional grazed foot or knee would bring tears, but Nanna Jean was there to wipe them away and tell us to get back out there. My life as a young boy was all about bare-foot fun and a free imagination. Nothing else mattered.

Our town hosted all types of weather, and as a child I embraced every aspect of nature, my home: the feel of bare feet on the earth, the sea breeze, salt air and lush green hills were my paradise. Freedom was a neighbourhood flush with kids, running, playing, falling down and getting up, outdoors from dawn to dusk.

Several playmates were always up for adventure and excitement. I biked around the streets, through the bush, and down steep, muddy hills with Hayden Scott, Tyler Coll and Ben Wallace, crashing and coming up laughing, no fears or worries.

My best friend was Lisa, the girl next door. We hung out together every day, running around or bike riding, building huts, popping tar bubbles and teasing the teenaged paperboy. The naughtiest, coolest line we could come up with was, 'A big apple crunch.' We'd stand bravely behind the protection of a fence, yelling, 'Hey, paper boy, you big apple crunch!' Lisa's mum Sandy would come storming over and tell us off for being so disrespectful.

I started school at Grey Main Primary, made friends easily, got into sport and had plenty of fun making trouble. It was a two-minute walk to school down an alleyway bounded by a tall fence. On the other side was a big German Shepherd who'd bark like mad whenever stones crunched in the alley. The dog scared the shit out of six-year-old me and I'd run as fast as I could down the alley and across the field to school.

I took up several sports and played every day: rugby, league, basketball, squash, cricket and swimming. I was shy and reserved, but sport gave me a desire to test how far I could go and I was always pushing myself. Sport brought out the best in me, and my cheeky sense of humour. I had energy to burn.

I was a sensitive kid. I had to *feel* things to understand them and to learn. If something didn't resonate with me, then it served no purpose. Running made sense because I *felt* it. I could be myself, at one with my thoughts, with no rules, no teachers telling me what to do, no Mum and Dad telling me off. I felt my heart beat, my breath go in and out. I loved my body and all I could get from it. Whatever I undertook, I did it 100 percent. That was the only way I could be or I lost my sense of purpose. I was strongest at running and was never one to walk a cross-country. I ran everywhere.

Early role models

Dad had a much tougher upbringing than I did. His father immigrated to New Zealand from the devastation of post-war Holland, hoping to start a new life for himself and his five children.

My grandfather was a tough man. He worked my father hard and beat him, although deep down I know he had a kind heart and loved his children. It was hard, raising his family single-handedly while trying to establish himself in a new country far from home.

Dad grew up in Whataroa, a small farming town near Franz Josef. His mother passed away when he was just two years old, so my grandfather sent Dad and his siblings away to Christchurch to be taught and raised by the nuns for six years. At 17 he left to find his way in the world. He took a job with the railways in Greymouth as an electrical apprentice and met Mum at a youth group event. We often tease Dad over how he managed to get a girl like Mum, saying she's an 'angel' and he's 'one lucky man', punching above his weight big-time.

I'm the oldest in our family, born when Dad was just 22. He was big, muscled, tough, the scariest man in the world with legs like tree trunks, who did press-ups while I rode on his back. He always wore a blue-checkered railways Swanndri, rugby shorts and boots.

Dad was a strong, rarely-seen presence in our home when I was growing up. He worked at the Kokiri meat works, then at the Spring

Creek coal mine. An electrician by trade, he took as much overtime as he could to provide for the family and put some away for a future lifestyle where he wouldn't have to work as hard. He came home late, tired, hungry and angry at the people he worked with, or frustrated over something that had happened during the day.

My grandfather's tough parenting had rubbed off on Dad, and as the oldest child and son, I frequently bore the brunt of his anger. We clashed and fought a lot yet still shared a love and deep respect for each other. I used to wish for another kind of father-figure in my life. I was far closer to Mum because she expressed so much love for me, my brother and sister.

One time I was crying for no memorable reason. Dad had had enough so he hit me hard with a bamboo stick – *whack, whack, whack* – saying, 'I'll give you something to cry about'. After that, I was often punished with the bamboo stick and Rachael would watch and cry. My mother was always there to wipe our tears afterwards, and I was definitely a mum's boy at heart. Dad's tough parenting provided me with good discipline and strength, but as a result of his harsh words and criticism I learned to hold back my tears and adopted the attitude that 'men don't cry'. This attitude would later change.

My favourite toy from an early age was a shovel. I carried it with me everywhere, even in my pram, resting it across my lap. Mum would get stuck in shop doorways as she tried to push me through.

When I was seven, Dad gave me the lawn mower to push around the yard. He wanted to see if I could handle it. The mower weighed a ton but I was determined to mow a row. I thank him to this day because cutting those lawns gave me a compulsion to push, to sweat, a craving to feel my heart hammering like a drum in my chest and the blood pulsing through my veins. The cut grass on a summer's day lit up my eyes and the smell became an addiction. It was the scent of nature and I felt it around me. To Mum's dismay I started mowing the lawns with bare feet so I could feel and smell the grass at the same time.

I loved proving that I could do it and showing Dad I was tough.

The mower taught me that if I pushed hard enough, I could achieve whatever I wanted, and that there was always an end to a job, pursuit, or challenge.

And I put that favourite toy to good use, too, shovelling the coal off with Dad. I was hooked, constantly mowing the lawns, shovelling coal and proving my strength but, to Dad's dismay, also getting in the way a lot.

Little did I know that this hard, physical work was building a base of body strength, the foundation for my running later on.

My brother Jake and my sister Rach

Rachael is two years younger than me and used to sneak into my bed during thunder storms. My job as an older brother was to comfort her and tell her everything was okay while she fell back to sleep beside me. My brother Jacob came along five years later. I really took on board 'bringing him up' – not that I had to. I just loved him so much. At school our teacher asked us to bring along a favourite toy, or something we loved, to talk about in front of the class. I was eight. Jake was only a few months old, but I took him as my 'show and tell'. I was so proud to have a baby brother. I taught Jake to walk. Every day I held his hand as he tottered down the hallway, one step at a time.

With Dad working six or seven days a week, Jake and I didn't get much quality time with him. I was the one who took the punishment Dad gave out. I didn't want my brother to endure it. Jake was my best mate.

Schoolboy working life

I inherited Dad's solid, hard-working habits and always had an after-school job. During school holidays, Dad took us to the farm at Whataroa where he grew up and we would help with the haymaking. I met up with my other cousins on Dad's side of the family: Dave,

Blair, Julia, Theresa, Geraldine and Ashleigh. I learned to drive tractors and stack hay from eight years onwards. On those hot summer days, after the work was done, I was allowed a 'shandy' (lemonade mixed with a bit of beer). At nine years old I felt like a real man drinking with the men. Having a 'beer' was a treat, one I bragged about to my mates back at school.

When I was 13 I had the hilliest paper route in town. It started at Freyberg Terrace, went over the Greymouth Hill and around the back side of town, finishing with Tindale Road and one final, steep hill. Mum drove the car on wet days while I ran the whole way. My heart and legs were getting stronger. I loved to run. I ran the six kilometres out to the Rangi Reserve and back. Not bad for a young fellow. Sometimes Reece Kennedy, my friend from next door, would join me on his bike. I loved being outdoors and was often at the skate park or out mountain biking up and down Power Station hill.

During the school holidays I worked at Mitre 10 hardware, sweeping the floor and crushing boxes, and at 15 I was employed at Southeran's Joinery to sweep and do deliveries, to glaze windows and help build kitchen units. The sweeping gave me a good workout, building up my arm and core muscles.

At secondary school I didn't take my running as seriously as the competitors from other secondary schools, so my placings at national competitions were not significant. I always did well in Greymouth, though, where my times met the New Zealand standard for my age group.

We ran barefoot down at ANZAC park. You could hear the sea from there, and see the beautiful Paparoa Range hulked up in the distance. There were little prickles in the grass. We dodged them when walking, but there was no way to avoid them when running. All of us kids complained to our parents about the prickles and the reply was, 'If you run fast enough you won't feel them.'

I see myself running on a hot summer day at ANZAC Park in Greymouth. It always felt like freedom to me, the cool breeze on my face, my friends around to laugh and race with. Running on the clean, freshly cut grass gave me a deep happiness that would stay with me for the rest of my life.

'Kick the butt!'

I first met Danny Spark at the Greymouth Athletic Club. He motivated and inspired me to get down and work hard at my running. He was famous for yelling at the kids, 'Kick the butt!' Although he wasn't a fully-fledged coach, Danny loved helping the kids and took a lot of time for us all. Danny favoured the Lydiard System (Arthur Lydiard was a New Zealand coach who triggered the 'jogging' boom) and had a real enthusiasm for encouraging and helping kids like me.

The Greymouth junior athletics were held each summer on a Saturday morning. On my first day I won the sprints and a couple of distance races. I can hear Danny's voice even now, yelling in the background, 'Kick the butt! Kick the butt!' When I hit the top of the bend, I'd hear, 'Kick the butt!' and find I still had some pace to run.

I played rugby for Blaketown and league for Suburbs and went on to make the West Coast teams in both sports, from the under-9 right through to the under-18. At a young age I was active and training hard, even though I developed later than most other boys. Speed had always been my greatest asset and they started to beat me in the sprints. However, my distance running improved. I gritted my teeth and hung in there for the win. I was doing well. When I ran I thought of nothing but the finish line as I breathed the air deep into my lungs, and no matter how long the race, I was in tune with my body.

High school days

I attended Grey High School, worked hard at my subjects, enjoyed athletics and playing rugby, league and basketball. We had plenty of fun as well. One day, my friend Nathan McEwen and I took all the chrome door handles off the Social Studies and English blocks and buried them in the garden. We later found out they were worth a couple of thousand dollars and weren't discovered until we had left the school.

A favourite morning tea activity was to go over the road to the New World supermarket, buy bags of apples and throw them at each other over the basketball court. Apples all over the place, and more than a few fights unfolded.

I made good friends at Grey High, and we got to know each other better through playing community sports. My best mate Hamish was a country kid. He loved sport, hard work and having a laugh as much as I did. We played for the same rugby league team, the Waro Raku Hornets. A big fellow, soft-spoken, Hamish played in the second row, one of the best physical players we had. At an end of year break-up, our under-16s shared the prize-giving with the seniors, and large quantities of beer and spirits were consumed by all. It was Hamish's first time drinking in town so we made the most of it. At 15 we thought we could drink as much as we wanted without consequences.

My mate Nathan also played for Waro Raku and we decided to take off, get into mischief and have a laugh. We forgot to tell Hamish. Come 11 pm, he thought I'd gone home. He walked down the road to my place, drunk and staggering. It was my sister's birthday that night and Mum was driving round town, dropping off her friends to their homes, when they saw Hamish wandering aimlessly on the footpath. Mum pulled over and said, 'Is that you, Hamish?' One of the girls in the car yelled out, 'Man, you're drunk!' Not realising who was in the car, Hamish pulled the finger and yelled out, 'Fuck you!' Harsh words for the politest man I know. Alcohol brings out the best in us. When Hamish got to my house he tripped at the doorway and his head went through the glass ranch slider. Dad thought someone was breaking into the house until he saw this big bear lying on the driveway with the broken trophy he'd just won: 'Best Forward for the Season'. Dad picked him up, carried him inside and put him on my bed. I came home to a smashed window and Hamish's vomit all over my room. We've been the best of mates ever since.

'Fight to get the job done.'

I left school at 17, in spite of my dream to be a physiotherapist since I'd passed NCEA levels one and two quite comfortably. My dad pulled me out at year 12, sick of getting phone calls from the school. With far too much energy, I was having a lot of fun and disrupting the class. I applied for two jobs, one at the Spring Creek coal mine, and the other at Electronet Services as a line mechanic. Electronet offered first. Looking back, I'm very grateful because that job suited me well. I started work with my friend Brogan Thomson. At knock-off time, Brogz and I got together to talk about all we'd accomplished that day as two apprentices.

It was hard work, outdoors every day in all weathers – rain, high winds, snow and hail – driving around the Coast rigging up lines and working with a gang of tough men. The men were hard on boys like me. The only way to gain their respect was to work twice as hard: dig the best holes I could as fast as I could, stand a pole and carry ladders through the bush. I learned to fell trees with a chainsaw, rig up power lines, and of course make a decent cup of tea.

I joined a gang with Tony Fearn and Bob Bostwick and we worked together for years. They showed me the value of hard work and reward. Bobby was a role model and father figure – funny, strong, kind and caring. Both he and Tony taught me anything I wanted to know. I learned quickly and they often trusted me to do technical jobs by myself. At 19, I was soon organising jobs of my own.

Once, Bob and I were together on the top of a hill in Blacks Point just out of Reefton. We had to fly two poles, and two cross-arms (an 'H' structure) was being flown in by helicopter. Bob said, 'Josh, this is going to be a difficult job and we'll have to fight to get it done.' He was right. It was difficult and we struggled with the cross-arms and poles, to join everything up. It was just the two of us, alone on the ridge in the middle of the bush.

Tony, a.k.a. 'Fearny', and Bob were both great to me. We became a little family on Truck 36 and got all the big jobs.

I was training hard too. Bob and Fearny often dropped me off at

Stillwater, 16 km out of Greymouth, and I'd run home. A hard day's work followed by intensive training was exhausting. I loved it.

Bob died when I was 20. I loved him like a father. His wife, Dot, gave me the hard hat that was on his coffin and she said, 'You were his boy.' I've never forgotten those words. Thank you, Dot. Bob used to say, 'Fight to get the job done.' Those words resonate with me today. Thank you, Bobby.

My friend Kieran died not long after. I had a beer with Kieran on the Wednesday and by Friday he was dead. He was welding at work, a spark went astray and there was an explosion. It was a terrible shock, losing one of my best mates at such a young age. From Kieran's death I learnt that life was short, and that I needed to make the most of the opportunities it presented me.

The Coast way

At the time I started working, I was enjoying my running more than ever and taking it seriously. Glenn Gibb, 'Gibby', was our next-door neighbour and the local 'I-do-everything' man. A coal miner by trade, Gibby was another alternative father figure of mine. He was a former New Zealand rugby league rep and loved his fitness.

Living next door, he often came by my house and we'd go for a run uphill and around the streets of Greymouth, or over the Point Elizabeth track. His enthusiasm, hard work and energy were contagious and I ran with him regularly. He pushed me.

'Yo, Josh, let's do it, mate, let's go running!' We even ran on Christmas Day. I thought this man was mad and I was right, but Gibby was awesome and he taught me so much. His kindness, caring and advice never stopped. He did everything he could to help, motivating me to run, to dig deep and push. This was the Coast way. I was on Gibby's page, doing everything the best I could at 100 miles an hour.

At 17, I wanted to take my running to the next level and asked New Zealand marathon legend and local identity Dave McKenzie to coach me. Dave was a former champion of both the Boston and New

Zealand marathons. He agreed to take me on.

I was soon out on 90-minute runs with the legendary Eddie Gray. Eddie was a former 10 km and New Zealand Cross Country Champion. He'd won a bronze medal at the World Cross Country Championships in 1971, and together we ran along parts of the Coast Road tracks that very few people knew about. Along the way he told me about the coal mining history at Runanga township, and the coal mines of Strongman, Ruanui and 10 Mile. I enjoyed every minute of our time together. I respected Eddie's wisdom and knowledge and was always picking his brains about the training he'd done at my age, absorbing as much as I could.

Ruth Croft was a local girl boarding over in Christchurch at Rangi Ruru girls' college. She ran with us out on the Coast Road during the school holidays. Ruth and I became good friends and often in summer we'd head to the Brunner Mine site bridge to jump in and swim. Nothing better after a run in the hot sun with the sweat dripping off you. We trained hard, and rewarding ourselves with a bathe in the river became our tradition.

Being coached and mentored by two legends inspired me to work hard and do well. I wanted to restore Greymouth's running reputation so I became passionate about the sport and our local history. I trained six days a week, worked full-time, and was addicted to cutting up firewood with Hamish. We went into the bush together, felling trees, ringing and splitting the wood for friends and family, selling a few loads here and there. Work and cutting firewood built my strength. I never needed to go to the gym. My body grew strong. I was lean, tough, determined, passionate and motivated. I wanted to win gold sometime at the New Zealand Championships and wear the Silver Fern on my chest at the Commonwealth Games. Since I was 13, that had been my ultimate life goal.

Dave was setting me up, building a base. I trained well and began competing in Christchurch at the under-19 races, winning the 5 km and placing in the 800 m and 1500 m. Jack O'Connor was a former New Zealand 400 m hurdle champion with a speed background.

Dave asked him to provide me with speed sessions. Dave looked on while Jack drew up the plan. The miles became speed-based and I became fast.

I won the under-19 Canterbury 1500 m and 800 m champs (2006 and 2007) and broke the West Coast record for the 800m, beating the top-ranked New Zealand Junior Jake Coom. Jake and I went on to become good friends.

The following season (2008), at 20 years old, I entered the Senior Men's division, won the 800 m Canterbury title and placed well in the 1500 m, booked a place in the New Zealand Senior Men's Canterbury Team, and broke the West Coast Senior Men's record for the 800 metres.

I then travelled to Auckland for the New Zealand Senior Athletic Champs, scheduled to compete in the 800 m and 1500 m. The 800 m was the focus. I was a fresh, confident 20-year-old, a typical first-timer with little idea of what to expect.

For my 800 m heat, Jack told me that if the pace was slow at the first 300 m I should just take off from the pack and take the race to them, stay out of trouble and finish comfortable. It was slow, and I went from 600 m, gapping the field by 15 m. I had the lead until the finish line. I was still fresh and had qualified for the final. I'd stayed out of the pack, out of the way and, most of all, out of trouble. The final was the following evening and my goal was to stay on the shoulder of current New Zealand champion Tim Hawkes. I kicked out too early with 320 m to go and he caught me, beating me over the line by less than half a metre. I finished a close second but still ecstatic at the placing. Jack ran over and hugged me, so proud. All the hard work had paid off. I ran my best, gave it my all, and could not have been happier. Finishing second at my first Senior Men's Champs and receiving my medal filled me with pride. It confirmed to me that hard work over talent was what it took to achieve my goals.

I'd trained while holding down a full-time job, put Greymouth running back on the map, and honoured the legacy of Dave and Eddie. I knew that if I moved to Christchurch and trained with others I would be hard to beat. My running career was just starting. It had all come together: the training with Eddie and Ruth on the Coast Road hills in all kinds of weather, the speed work with Jack, the miles with Dave, the encouragement from Gibby, working those 10- to12-hour days and cutting firewood with Hamish. I was ready to run fast and faster, and knew what I was capable of. I wanted to win my first New Zealand title and represent my country at the Commonwealth Games.

Disappointment

I wanted that gold medal at the New Zealand Athletic Championships, but a diagnosis of glandular fever meant time off from training and so no competing in 2009. In 2010 I was diagnosed with vestibular neuritis, a severe middle ear infection. I was dizzy, drained, tired easily and had only two months of preparation before the Championships that year. I came second in the 800 m event at the New Zealand Champs in Christchurch and received another silver medal. I was disappointed because ill health had impacted my training and I knew I could otherwise have won that race. Next year will be my year, I thought.

I left Greymouth to live in Christchurch so I could focus more on running. I shared a house with Jake Coom and worked at Mainpower as a powerline mechanic out in Rangiora. The work was easier than with Electronet. Better hours, less stress, more men on the job and no fighting with the rain and dense bush. The boys I worked with were great. They often let me leave the job site early to start running towards home, picking me up an hour later on their way through.

I was training twice a day, eating well, had given up alcohol and my body was humming like never before. I was fast, fit and happy with how things were progressing.

Don Grieg became a valued friend and mentor. He was an ex-New Zealand representative, one of our elite marathon runners. Dave and Jack were still my coaches. Don joined us at QE2 stadium, holding a stopwatch, calling my split lap times as I completed a workout, and telling me what I was doing right or wrong. I was in the best form of my life, and took second place in the 800 m at the Capital Classic in Wellington with a time of 1 minute 51 seconds and minimal speed work. Don and Jack were sure I was on track to take gold at the New Zealand Champs, on target for a sub 1.50 (running under one minute and 50 seconds for the 800 m) as I was in the form of my life!

In September 2010 Christchurch was hit by the first of many earthquakes. My flat was badly damaged so I moved in with running mate Dave Ridley. Work and training were going well. I exercised in the morning, worked hard all day, then ran and trained at night. All of the running over the Coast Road hills, the Port Hills, and the speed sessions with Jack and Don were paying off.

There were still days however when I asked myself, 'Why the fuck am I doing this running?' I ran in the pissing-down rain and snow on the Port Hills. Some days I had to stop and take a shit in the bush. I had no social life. Then I'd remind myself of the purpose behind this pain, the joy of achieving what I set out to accomplish, the reward of being the best 800 m runner I could be. I was in the form of my life and the New Zealand 800 m gold medal was in my sights.

I was out for the daily jog around Hagley Park with my training partner Andrew Davidson. We were chatting happily as usual when my weak ankle rolled over a tree root and lightning pain shot up my leg. I dropped to the ground and swore in agony and rage, at the world, at my stupid self. Andrew thought I was swearing at him, then his face changed as he realised what had happened. I told him I'd be okay: 'You run on, man. I'll sort myself out.' When he'd gone, I started to weep as I saw my New Zealand title hope vanishing for the year. I limped, head down, to the Avon River to soak the swollen ankle in cool water. Seven weeks before the Champs, I'd torn a ligament and chipped a bone in my right ankle. I pushed hard to recover, but the injury would not heal so I was forced to pull out. Again.

Anger, frustration, disappointment. The day I pulled out, I punched a tree outside the flat, over and over, tearing the bark off it, the broken skin on my fist bleeding down my arm and onto the footpath. I'd moved from home to Christchurch to make a go of my running and get the gold medal I wanted with such passion, and now the opportunity was lost. All my hard work ruined with this one stupid ankle injury. I went to my room, sat on the floor and cried alone, shedding tears about all the unpaid work I'd put in, and the sacrifices I'd made by not seeing friends and family. I felt I'd let down Dave, Jack, Don and the Greymouth community who had put so much time and effort into me. I'd tried my best and it had all come apart. I was so close to achieving my ultimate dream and it was taken from me, just like that. It was a disappointment I struggled with for years to come.

Then came 22nd February 2011. I was in Riccarton Mall, buying some new running shoes. The building began to shake with incredible force. I'd never felt so vulnerable before, like being on a boat on the rough waters of the Pacific Ocean. The building shook and rolled, glass broke and fell. People were screaming, dazed and running in terror. The city was in absolute chaos. As I drove back to my flat the road rose and fell beneath the car, like being on my surfboard paddling out over the waves. I was relieved to find my flat still standing with only a few cracks in the wall. I went around to the neighbours to see if they were okay. One old lady was just sitting motionless and crying in her living room chair, shaken and shocked. I brought her to our flat, comforted her and made her some tea. Seeing the city of Christchurch in ruins put into perspective the anger and disappointment over my stupid injury. Our city was badly damaged that day, and many people lost their lives. I was alive with just a sore foot.

It was a life-changing time, not only for Christchurch, but for me too. My body would not recover from my injury and I wasn't sure why. I had to face the reality that there would be no New Zealand Champs or gold medal for me.

The Lake Brunner

My body needed time to heal so I decided to have a complete break and go overseas with Brogan and Nathan, travel for six to eight months, then return home and give my running another go. The trip would give me the chance to fulfil some dreams and adventures. We all wanted UK visas but I didn't intend to stay there, preferring to get my skydiving ticket in Spain, and then go to Nepal Base Camp on my own. The visa would be a backup in case I needed it.

I moved back to family in Greymouth, shaken by the quakes, limping on my ankle and deeply disappointed. Still, I had the overseas travel to look forward to, so was content enough with life. I went back to Electronet for the two months before I flew out. I was exhausted by the end of each work day. I was sweating more than usual, and sleeping longer. I thought it was my body fighting a cold or maybe my foot was slowly healing.

I entered the Lake Brunner bike race, a 130 km loop, my 'last hurrah' before going overseas. The race is a major sporting event for Greymouth and I thought I'd be able to do it off the back of my training without much impact on the injured ankle.

My Uncle Kev is a competitive bastard and he said, 'You gotta beat all those cycling boys, eh Josh? They're soft. Show 'em what runners are capable of!'

'Yeah okay,' I said, 'I'll do that, mate, we'll show them!'

Race day was cold and wet. I started out well with Uncle Kev's words in my mind. I was in the lead pack for the first three km, pushing hard, and then I started to fade and halfway through the course, I was exhausted.

I collapsed at the Ivy Bay turnoff, seeing stars. I thought, What the fuck is going on? Get back on that bike, pick yourself up and keep going! I was shaking with fatigue, dizzy and struggling to breathe. Something wasn't right. My body was a machine, highly tuned, nothing could break me and I wasn't used to failure. I wondered if the glandular fever was coming back. I felt almost drunk. I was too confused to be angry or upset.

Being young and dumb I kept pushing, thinking maybe I was low on sugar. Anger kicked in – about not competing at the Champs and now failing at a bike ride – and kept me going. I said to myself, You're not going to fucking pull out of this, Josh. Fucking ride that bike otherwise you'll never hear the end of it from Uncle Kev.

I talked to myself, using the visualisation techniques that were an integral part of my training and that motivated me through the difficult days. I pictured myself pedalling to the finish line, then in bed resting, sleeping and healing. I kept saying to myself, Come on, Josh, come on, get to Moana, take a rest, this is only short-term pain. Finish the fucking race. At Moana, I staggered into the shop. I wanted sugar. I had no money and begged them to give me a can of Coke and a chocolate bar. I sat out front, chewed the Snickers, drank the Coke and told myself, Finish this fucking race, Josh.

I pedalled and pedalled. My head drooped over the handlebars and I was pedalling so slowly everyone was passing me. I was fading. I had never hit the wall so hard. My legs became bricks, then lead weights. I knew the landmarks coming up so set myself little goals: Ruth's place, her dad's trucking company, then Stillwater, followed by the Brunner Bridge where Ruth and I swam, Kaita, and finally Greymouth.

'Please finish,' I said aloud. 'You can do it, you can get there. Please, Josh, get there, then you can rest. Get to the corner. You're on a straight now. This is easy, keep pedalling and pushing. You have run to Greymouth from here, so keep going.'

My head was still drooping, my eyes were rolling back and I didn't know what was wrong with me. I was nearly the last to finish. Uncle Kev had left by then, thinking I'd pulled out. I collapsed over the line and vowed never to ride a fucking bike again.

After the Lake Brunner race, I stayed in bed and slept for five days. I had night sweats so severe I woke up thinking I'd pissed the bed. My face in the mirror was white. When I went to the doctor, they said I must have had mild hypothermia. They didn't do any tests and said I'd be okay in a few weeks.

Up until that bike race, life had seemed fair. Sure, there were always two sides to it, opposites that belong together – laughter and tears, sadness and fun, good and bad, up and down… Things were never perfect, always switching about, but on the whole, life was fair. As I lay in bed, so exhausted I could only get up to eat a little and use the toilet, I thought about my life and my future, grateful for what I had achieved, but also deeply disappointed that my goals and hard work hadn't been realised as I'd expected. I was ready to leave New Zealand for a better place than this, where I could forget about the past year. I'd rest and heal, then come back to my running with more fight inside. Looking back, I know it was my mind that needed to change, not the place where I was.

In a few days, I'd be flying out on my big OE. I had to fight off this whatever-it-was. I had so much to look forward to.

I had no idea how sick I was. I was dying and I didn't have a clue.

14 May 2011

It was a cold, rainy morning. I woke up feeling confused, with no idea what was happening to my body. My left eye was swollen. I felt dizzy and dazed. I went to the hospital. There, they tried unsuccessfully to reduce the swelling, then sent me home with antibiotics.

I grew worse as the day progressed. I was running myself a cup of water at the sink when I passed out. Jacob was home and he rang my Auntie Irene who was a nurse. She said, 'Get him up to that hospital *now*.' When I came around, the left side of my face was even more swollen, but it was a few hours before Mum came home and could take me up there. As we sat in the waiting room, I kept telling her, 'Something's not right, Mum. Something's not right.' She rubbed my back and comforted me as I cried softly, angry and frustrated to the core. I was torn, wanting answers, but also wanting badly to leave! It was Friday and I was due to fly to Thailand on Sunday. They kept me in overnight, gave me more antibiotics and finally did blood tests. I awoke the next day feeling a little better.

PART TWO
CANCER

He who has a why
to live can bear
almost any how.

— FRIEDRICH NIETZSCHE

I LAY in bed in the open, empty room: four walls, no windows, six beds and only two patients. The other was an old man who looked as though he might be on his last legs. The room echoed with death. What the fuck was I doing in hospital? I was meant to be flying out with my mates tomorrow.

As lunchtime approached, Mum and Dad came up to visit, soon followed by my Uncle Blue. It was nice to have them to talk to, and to eat the decent food they'd brought in. Uncle Blue's a hardened old bastard with a heart of gold. He slouched against the wall and gave me shit about being there. As ever, he made me laugh and helped shift the negative thoughts.

Mum and Dad were standing at the foot of my bed looking anxious when Dr Sharp approached with the news that would change my life for ever. He didn't beat around the bush. He said the blood tests showed that I had leukaemia.

Leukaemia? It sounded like a made-up word.

'What the hell is that?' I groaned.

'Well, Josh, it's cancer in your blood,' he said.

'How did that happen? I'm 23, one of the fastest track runners in New Zealand. I'm going away with my friends tomorrow.'

'No, Josh, you're not going anywhere. You're going to the Bone Marrow Unit in Christchurch for seven months of treatment.'

All I heard was, *Josh, you are going to get fucked up, full of chemo.*

In that moment, the dark gloom of the day outside swept into the room. By this time my good mate Nathan had turned up. He and my family were in tears. Nathan hugged me and Uncle Blue kept saying, 'No, no, no', shaking his hands wildly in the air.

The news wasn't sinking in. What the fuck was going on? Was I dying? I sat up straight in bed and looked around. Or was this an elaborate joke?

The tears, sadness and pain in the room told me it was no joke. I closed my eyes to shut out those whose crying howled through the room. I tried to find the place in my mind where I belonged. In nature, calm and peaceful. I opened my eyes and the reality of the 'cancer' word hit me like a cold stone wall. I looked at Mum, my beautiful, loving Mum, who stood beside my bed with tears rolling down her face. Not tears of sadness, but fearful tears that were too hard to watch.

The harsh Greymouth rain poured down outside, and inside her tears were like a flooded river with deadly rapids; they spoke for the feeling in the room.

I looked around as the raw emotion of everyone in the room unfolded in slow motion. It was puzzling that a simple word could produce such intense reaction. I felt the sadness, but didn't understand it. All I said was, 'Don't cry, Mum. I'll be okay. I'll fight. It's just leukaemia.'

Welcome to the cancer world

How naïve I was. I had no idea what I was in for or what this diagnosis meant.

I said to the doctor, 'Well, what are we waiting here for? Take me to Christchurch, replace my blood, problem solved.'

'It's not that simple,' he said.

He was talking about 'chemotherapy' and 'medical treatments' and I was still thinking 'sprained ankle', a bit of this 'chemo' stuff, an ice pack or two and I'd be away again. I had no idea that my life was going to change from that day, in every way possible – mentally, physically and spiritually – forever. No teacher in the world could tell me what I was going to learn about the human body and about myself.

As the doctor talked, things began making sense. When he told me I had only 40 percent of my red blood cells, I understood my struggle on the bike ride. There wasn't enough oxygenated blood going to my tissues and organs for them to function properly. The white blood cell count was out of control. I had far too many.

Still in Grey Hospital, I had the first of many blood transfusions, a bag of blood into each arm. My hands lay palms up; I couldn't bend my elbows. As the blood flowed through, I thought, since it's a blood cancer, why don't they just drain my blood and re-infuse me with new blood?

My education about the human body was starting, knowledge and understanding that would blow me away. Life is learning. I meant to take in as much as I could from this situation so I asked questions. My theory about replacing my blood was rejected. Things didn't work that way. The problem lay with my 'cell factory', the bone marrow. It wasn't producing red and white blood cells correctly and so my whole immune system was out of order.

Confusion gave way to anger because my travels *and* my running were all gone. Why me? Why now? The tears came then. How was I going to get through this? How could I win this race?

I didn't sleep that night as the monitor clicked over, and new blood or fluids were put up every few hours. I was weak and tired but my mind was racing. I studied the blood running into my arms. How the fuck did cancer get in there? I wanted to fix this problem myself, but I knew nothing. I had to trust that the doctor's information, and the medications he was giving me, would sort this out. I needed to find as much information as I could. Thoughts ran through my head, all night long. What the fuck was going on? What was this? Was it a joke? I was so fit and strong, people like me didn't get cancer. I was confused, angry, frightened. My world was falling apart.

The question kept arising: Was I going to die?

There was a smell in the room. It lingered like a stray dog, following me, tormenting me. To this day, the smell reminds of all I've endured: the pungent stink of pure alcohol. Wiped on my skin before a needle was inserted into the vein, or used to clean my sterile room, that smell became the stench of pain and makes me sick to the stomach even now.

The doctor told me what I could expect during chemotherapy. I would lose my hair, for one thing. That was the least of my worries because he said it would grow back. The prospect of being cooped up in a hospital room was far worse, when all I wanted was to run and be free.

I could forget running out on the Coast Road with Ruth and Eddie, all my track races, a good, hard day at work, cutting and splitting firewood with Hamish or swimming at Brunner Bridge. All I had to look forward to was the South Island Bone Marrow Unit in Christchurch. Welcome to the world of cancer, Josh.

The biggest race of my life was still to come and I had no idea how extreme it would be. Suffering, agony and pain. Life was just starting.

The Bone Marrow Unit

The sun shone the next morning: typical Greymouth, cold and wet one day, beautiful the next. I stared out the hospital window with the bright sun on my face. I closed my eyes tight, saw the red behind my eyelids, soaked it up like never before. It made me smile and for a brief moment I was calm, felt no fear. Then I saw the needles in my arms and realised what lay ahead today: The Bone Marrow Unit in Christchurch where I would find out more about my cancer and treatment. With my eyes closed, I pictured another place, far away. I was running out on the Coast Road where the crash of ocean waves and the green lush bush filled my senses with utter joy. I'd practised visualising when preparing for a big race, seeing where I wanted to be in the race and when I'd start sprinting for the finish. Now the race was my life, so daily, even hourly, I pictured myself healthy again and doing the things I loved. Visualisation could take me from the real world to where I wanted to be, and for brief moments I could create my own Garden of Eden and feel goodness flood my body. Then I'd open my eyes and move on.

Mum and Dad drove me the three hours to Christchurch, from the west of the South Island to the east. Jake and Rachael came too. Few words were spoken on the way. As we crossed Arthur's Pass, the heavy grey clouds reflected the mood in the car.

I longed to be on the top of that hill, or up in those clouds, anywhere but in this mess. I thought about my siblings. Jake was my best mate and I loved Rachael. I'd always been their role model and protector, the oldest and strongest and now I had cancer. I felt weak and pathetic, though I needed to stay brave and strong for Jake because he looked up to me. He was only fifteen. I had to show him how good life was, and encourage him to embrace every moment of it.

My head was buzzing the whole way with frantic thoughts of death. I stayed calm on the outside, trying to show I was brave. Inside was turmoil. I had no idea what the treatment would be like. I didn't know anyone who'd received chemotherapy apart from my former boss Kent Martin who told me a little of his experience. He'd suggested I write a daily diary to help pass the time.

I had so many questions. Would I be in a room full of other people? How long would the treatment last? Would it hurt? Could I ever run again, or travel? How did this happen and why? How advanced was the cancer? I wondered, over and over, like a stuck record: would I die?

The drive to Christchurch was the longest journey of my life.

Safe havens

We'd been told about Ranui House, accommodation near Christchurch Hospital for families supporting long-term patients. This took a weight off my parents' shoulders as my family wanted to be with me for the duration of my treatment. My place would be in the Bone Marrow Unit.

Christchurch Hospital was huge, compared to Greymouth Hospital, a maze of corridors and rooms. Adrenaline had kicked in, in this unknown setting, and I found the strength to walk – like a scared kid – at Mum's side. Looking for the Unit, I felt rushed and worried. After a lot of, 'Excuse me, do you know where the Bone Marrow Unit is?' we found my new home.

A nurse took me to my room, an isolation facility the size of a bedroom with double air-vented entry doors, a toilet, shower and sink, and a large window with a view of the park. This tiny new room was to become my safe haven.

There was that smell again, from Greymouth Hospital, the alcohol. On top of that was an odour of dryness, kind of like cardboard, a smell of nothing, devoid of life, fun or colour. How would I handle being locked away from the trees, the fresh, soft wind, the sun's warmth? The battle for my life would take place in locked-up isolation. This was prison and I felt despair like never before.

I had already decided to fight this cancer alone. I didn't want my family to grow any more worried. I hated to see them looking so lost, scared and confused. I hated all the attention I was getting, the panic I was causing. Shutting my family out of the situation would ease their stress. My middle name was Stubborn and my tagline was, 'I'll get this shit done by myself.' I was a strong man. I could handle it.

The reality was quite different. I was a lost little boy, trapped in a world where I didn't belong, one that would tear me apart and build me back into someone new. Once I was settled into the unit, I sent my family away to Ranui House. I told them everything was fine. I was managing this like a race: pushing up the hill, putting on my brave face, hurting so bad but never letting my opposition know.

My family, my opposition. I loved them but I excluded them and sent them away. I was frightened, alone, tired, angry. I was running this race by myself. In retrospect, I know they were my allies, my friends, the ones to help me. My attitude was all wrong. I hurt them with my dismissal and taking on this mountain by myself would nearly break me. But I had to learn that the hard way.

My new best friend: Mr. Hickman

I sat on the only chair, with a pile of papers and cancer information in my lap. CML, AML, ALL, CLL. There was more than one type of leukaemia and which one did I have?

Then the tea lady came in, shrieking, 'Menu! Menu!'

'I don't have it,' I replied.

'Well, you'd better get it done or else you won't have anything to eat,' she said.

It wasn't long before the doctors arrived and I met my specialist, Dr Peter Ganly. He gave me a rundown of what would happen over the next week: more blood tests, a Hickman line inserted into my chest, a bone marrow biopsy, MRI and CT scans. What on earth was all this mumbo jumbo?'

A line in my chest? I didn't know they could do that. The doctor said the Hickman line would be my 'new best friend', saving me from a lot of needles. He explained that the line is a 'venous catheter inserted into your chest and into the subclavian vein just outside of your heart'.

Holy shit, I thought. This was just the start.

I calmed myself by thinking of my diagnosis as a race, the doctors as my coaches. I told myself to do what they said, do what I needed to get this done. This was a road block and I could get around it.

I closed my eyes and put all of my energy into visualising myself out of that isolation room and into 'my world' where I was free, happy, and running again in the open air with Ruth and Eddie along the beautiful Coast Road. I remembered how much I loved running over the tops of the Paparoas (the range of hills behind Greymouth), having travel adventures, and I reminded myself of the lifelong dreams I had yet to fulfil, of becoming a skydiver and getting to Everest Base Camp.

Visualising would become a daily practice, every hour of every day. I pictured myself in full health, doing the things I loved, being strong and happy again. In my mind I was free – not in this tiny room and not with cancer, chemo and pain. Cancer and the treatment might take my physical health, but there was no way they'd take my mind or so I hoped.

45

Mr Hickman did become my new best friend. The line was inserted into my chest, blood was drawn from it for testing, and through it I was given transfusions, saline, and antibiotics for my swollen eyes. This was far easier on my veins – no needles, no pain.

This would be a breeze now. This Hickman was awesome.

Or so I thought. It was bad enough smelling the alcohol in the room, but now I tasted it. The Hickman line was cleaned with pure alcohol, so every day I received a shot of it. The taste was vile. It burned my throat and made me dry-retch. I told myself I'd never drink alcohol again.

The next day I was to have a bone marrow biopsy to determine what kind of leukaemia I had and how significant the cancer was. I was introduced to Nic, a lovely nurse and my primary caregiver. She outlined the procedure. They were going to stick a big needle in my hip and suck some bone from it.

'Holy shit, for real?' I said.

'Yes,' Nic said, 'but they give you gas to help ease the pain.'

'Okay, no problem. I'll make the most of the gas.'

I lay down on my bed with the gas mask over my face, breathing deep and enjoying it as best I could. The doctor began the procedure. I felt a small prick as the needle went through my skin. Five seconds later it drilled into my hip.

'Fuck!' I yelled.

As I took more gas to ease the pain, the distant view of Hagley Park started to fade and my eyes rolled back. I smiled to myself. Was this the worst they could do? Fuck cancer! Then the doctor began extracting the marrow and the gas didn't even touch the sides of the pain. I'd taken too much gas the first time so they took it away and I had to endure the procedure without it. I swore, never again.

'That's just the beginning,' the doctor said. 'You'll need one of these after every cycle of chemo, once a month.'

The results came through and Dr Peter told me I had acute myeloid leukaemia, AML.

'Okay,' I said slowly, feeling confused, 'What does that involve?'

'It's a very fast-growing and aggressive form of leukaemia,' said Peter. 'We want to start treatment now.'

Peter offered participation in an international trial to see which combinations of chemo drugs were most effective, and hopefully gain a complete remission of AML. I accepted. I'd receive three different chemotherapy drugs in combination. The cancer was present in my central nervous system too, so three times a week I would have lumbar punctures. A needle full of chemo drugs would be inserted through the base of my spine and into the cerebro-spinal fluid. All of this would start the following day.

I would spend a month at a time in isolation, receiving treatment. The room was small like a shoe box, had a double ventilated door system and a Hepa filter which filtered the air in the room, removing small particles and reducing the risk from mould and fungal spores that were potentially bought into the room. All this safety would reduce my risk of infection. After the month, I could leave for ten days, then return to do it all again. The treatment would take about seven months.

After Peter left, Nic set up my daily doses of blood, antibiotics and fluids and sat down with me.

'The chemo will make you very sick,' she said, 'so I'll give you pills to reduce the nausea.'

'No worries,' I said. 'I've had plenty of hangovers before.'

Chemotherapy

My first day of chemo went well at first, with no immediate nausea. That night I threw up suddenly and violently, all over the sink and myself.

This wasn't like any hangover I'd ever had. The taste of vomit in my mouth was so vile it made me feel even sicker. I thought I was throwing up my stomach. I took a tablet to help me sleep. I needed rest because another round was scheduled for the next day.

The first cycle was the hardest of the four I'd receive. I had a continual fever and developed rigors, whole-body shakes, feeling cold and sweating so hard it felt like I'd wet the bed. Icebreaker thermals absorbed the sweat, so I didn't need the sheets changed so often. I developed a 'leukaemic eye' and couldn't see out of my left eye.

My body felt tangled up. I was a weak, exhausted mess. Worse than a hard training session. No comparison.

The ongoing, intense chemotherapy lowered my neutrophils. (Neutrophils are our main infection and pathogen fighter.) The 'neutropenia' meant that my immune system had become dangerously weak. I had to stay in isolation so I wouldn't pick up any viruses or bacteria. The small room became my safe house.

As course followed course, my body shrank and I grew weaker every day. The anti-nausea drugs had little effect. I was used to home-cooked meals – slow-roasted lamb and fresh fish. Now I struggled to swallow the food provided. My body craved salt and sugar, so for breakfast I'd make my own toast with the toaster in my room, and spread four tablespoons of butter on each slice.

Every day the doctors came in to tell me what else they'd found out about the cancer. Dr Ganly told me I had these different markers: inversion 16 chromosome, positive for FLT 3 protein and core binding factor. I just looked at him, like a new apprentice starting the job wide-eyed, nodding yes, over and over, with no idea what was said to me. These markers meant my prognosis was not great. Fear was settling in. I bought some books to understand what this leukaemia was all about, to try and ease my mind. I wanted to know everything I could and Dr Google was a great tool. I was so weak and sick, I hated my situation. One week into treatment I started to cry, I mean really cry. Not little tears, but big tears of hate, anger and anguish. I hated myself for becoming sick and was so fearful of the weak, fragile person I'd become. I looked at myself in the mirror and said, 'You're a loser.' The life I knew and respected had been taken away from me.

Dad had always told me that men don't cry. I'd lock myself in the bathroom with my pump beeping outside and I'd cry, tears rolling down my cheeks like the Grey River in flood. I'd hide so the nurses couldn't see me. They always knew, though, because they heard my cries of despair.

I'd spend about 15 distressed minutes in there, crying, hating my life and what had happened to me, searching for a reason. Then I'd pull myself together and come out of the bathroom in a state of complete exhaustion.

I tried to picture myself running again. This had always worked before. But I was too weak now and it gave me no reassurance or comfort at all. I lay on my bed exhausted, sad and frustrated, desperate to leave the little box-like room.

My mum, brother and sister visited and tried to lighten my mood. They were always so sad and worried, though, and it made me angry. I made a rule: NO CRYING IN THIS ROOM. I took my anger and frustration out on my family. I didn't know who I was, or what I'd become.

My body grew weaker and my hair fell out. I barely coped with the pain of the bone marrow biopsies. Once the needle was inserted, I squeezed my eyes tight, trying to breathe through the pain, though small tears rolled down my cheeks. I breathed deep on the gas, wanting to pass out, which I did on occasion. After the procedure it would feel as though I'd been kicked in the lower back with steel-cap boots. Sometimes I didn't think I could take any more.

The chemo made my stomach shrink and hurt. The toxic chemo drugs had stripped the stomach lining. My nurses put up a big silver bag of liquid nutrients and hooked it into my Hickman line so the food went directly into my blood stream and not into my stomach.

I was sound asleep one afternoon when excruciating stomach pain woke me. This new agony was on a par with the bone marrow biopsies.

Pain after pain. I yelled and cried. My nurse Carol gave me IV morphine and then injected medicine directly into my stomach. The pain would not go. When she came back at 3 am with the fifth needle, I told her to fuck off, I didn't want her stupid shit because it wasn't working.

The nights were long. I wrote in my diary.

3 am in a hospital toilet bent over with your hands on your head and tears flowing. Outside the door is your friend, a friend you don't want, a friend that you need, one you can't talk to. An IV pole full of fluids, morphine and nutrients to keep you from losing any more weight.

You ask yourself this question every time you're here: Why are you crying? Why the fuck are you crying, you soft cunt. Oh, that's right, you have cancer, you have acute myeloid leukaemia.

Reality sets in and the tears don't want to stop. It's night time, no one is around, no visitors or nurses until 6 am. This is the only time I can hide and let out what I don't want people to see. I let the tears flow so there are none left for tomorrow.

Why am I crying?

It's not the pain, or being stuck in this empty room that's like a cave. It's because my life is in the doctors' hands, it's in a bag hooked to a pole. The bag contains chemicals that destroy everything in my body, just like cancer does.

Cancer. I hate that word. Do I really have cancer? Surely not, you can't get cancer. I repeat this word I hate, over and over, and say, 'Yes Josh, you do have cancer.' The tears flow again, my fists get tight, my forehead sweats, a rage builds up like a bull being taunted.

At 3 am I realise how much I hate this fucking place, and I wonder what the future holds. I dwell on the past with plenty of 'I should have done this' or 'Why didn't I do this earlier?' The past swells up like a tidal wave, then crashes down and, like a wall of water, it's out of control, going everywhere at once with immeasurable power and fury.

Exhausted and spent, I come out of the bathroom, wheel my friend back to the bed, my thumbs whip the tears away. The clock ticks, repeats, tick, tick, tick, inescapable. I can't sleep. My mind is humming.

Another day starts tomorrow. More chemotherapy. I don't understand the last part of the word. Therapy. When I hear it, I think of good, therapeutic healing. At this point there is nothing 'healing' about it. My stomach has shrunk to the size of a walnut, the pain is too immense to fight. I tried for a day, so I know. I gave in and they hooked me to a morphine pump so I had pain relief 24/7.

I have a Hickman line in my chest so all these chemicals can be fed into my bloodstream. I have a love/hate relationship with it. I want it there because it means fewer needles jammed into my skin and veins, and the doses they give me are far too great for a small vein to handle. I hate it because it allows them to put these poisons into me. I know these treatments are 'killing the cancer' but they're also killing me.

I lived on IV morphine for a few days and the pain finally subsided. I felt so bad about the way I had spoken to Carol. She was leaving the nursing profession that week and I didn't want one of her last patients to have been such a rude one, so I wrote her a note and apologised for my behaviour. She laughed and said, 'Love, I've dealt with more shit than that.' I remember thinking there must be some very difficult people out there. The nurses were well used to it though. They had seen every type of patient, and all types of cancer, chemo and diagnosis. They were amazing people and far more than nurses to me. They were my mum, counsellor, coach, and most of all, friend. They saw me at my worst and at my best and all wanted me to get through this cancer shit.

I then developed haemorrhoids which caused swelling and an enlarged anus. My bum was so sore every time I needed to poo it felt as if I was shitting barbed wire. I'd wipe ever so gently, dabbing softly, but it still felt as if I was wiping with a handful of glass. It was horrible and I soon needed a shot of morphine before I could go to the toilet.

Support from the Coast

Friends and family visited and I fronted up to them as bravely as I could. I never told them much. I put on a humorous face, as if nothing was wrong. I couldn't talk about my deep feelings. I didn't want to burden people with my problems. I've always been independent and wanted to put my head down and get the job done so I could go back to running and live again. I bottled everything up and cried myself to sleep.

I was changing physically and losing the plot. Running and being physically strong and fit for work was easy compared to this shit. And it was total shit, every day. I slept, threw up, and was constantly in pain somewhere. I was angry and took much of this frustration out on Dad because he has the thickest skin I knew. Dad had dealt with shit at work, and he said to me, 'Josh, I take insults and compliments the same.' I feel sorry now and owe him a debt of gratitude because in the early days post-diagnosis, he was the only person I could unload on and speak words that weren't nice or decent. He knew I was venting my frustration and he didn't take it personally. This was his way of helping me.

I was grateful for my friends although some days seeing people was just too much. I existed in another world and they didn't know what to do or say. The look on their faces summed it up: they had no idea what I was going through. It was too hard and I understood why some of them didn't visit again.

'How's it all going, Josh?' they'd ask.

'Yeah, good,' was my standard reply.

Support came from surprising quarters. People I hadn't had much to do with over the years showed up, and kept showing up. The Greymouth community organised fundraisers and my workmates at Electronet shaved their heads in support. I felt humbled by their kindness, and overwhelmed by the attention, unable to hold up my side of the deal. I'd been one of the fastest runners in New Zealand, but now I was one of the slowest and sickest, and people were giving me all this stuff. Why? Deep down, I was grateful for the support but it spun me out and was hard to deal with.

I was collecting a medical benefit too because there was no way I could work and I had no idea when I'd be able to again. Being from a Coast family, I'd been raised with the ethic: 'You earn what you get.' When Dad said, 'Josh, you deserve this,' it helped me accept the generosity shown. When times get tough, the people of the Greymouth community are well known for their kind hearts and humble spirits. The support they showed taught me to accept help.

Two friends, Hayden Scott and Kurt Neilson, decided to do a fundraiser for me. By now I was so overwhelmed and humbled by what the Greymouth community had already done, I suggested they donate to child cancer. Both the boys wanted to bike from Christchurch to the West Coast, which was quite ambitious for two under-trained recreational sportsman. Kurt's aunty had passed away in the CTV building in the Christchurch earthquakes, so it would also be a memorial ride for her. They both set off in the early morning, eager for the arduous 245-km bike ride. This would be their 'coast to coast' and it would be quite a feat for two unseasoned boys.

I got a phone call halfway through the ride from Mason Cox who was their motivator. He handed me over to Hayden and Kurt. They both sounded the way I felt: absolutely exhausted, overwhelmed and unmotivated. Kurt said to me, 'We can't do it, JK.' I replied in a voice groggy from the morning dose of chemo, 'If you start something, you finish it. I know you can do it, boys!' Sure enough they got back on their bikes, pedalling hard over the steep mountains that divided the Coast from Canterbury. The boys received a police escort into Greymouth. I was very proud of them both. It's incredible what the body can achieve once the mind has a vision, goal or purpose.

Hamish, my best mate, was living in Christchurch and he came to visit most days, stopping by after work. His company was healing balm for me, his presence uplifting. He was the friend I needed. Sometimes we'd talk. Other visits he'd just sit while I fought the fatigue.

Ruth was attending university in the USA on a running scholarship. She flew back to see me and always picked me up and gave me a lot of shit. My mate Matty Harry would pop in and talk and laugh. Jake Coom came in too, bringing food and drinks, taking the piss out of me for my bald head and my lost pubic hair, armpit hair and eyebrows. I'd lost it all and he didn't let up.

My childhood friend Ben Wallace flew down from Wellington to tell me he'd survived 'man 'flu' so I'd have no problem beating cancer.

I loved a laugh, and the saying 'humour is the best medicine'. I couldn't agree more.

Either my sister or my mum stayed at Ranui House for the duration of my treatment. Rachael literally moved in there as my caretaker, bringing over meals and other items I asked for, taking good care of her big bro.

The search was on for a bone marrow donor. This was our back-up plan if I relapsed after the treatment. I remember when Rachael learned she was a potential match. How excited we were! My sister was the key. What a gift she could give me! Rachael was so proud because she believed she was my lifesaver who could help in a way no one else could.

However, ten days later we were told she wasn't a match. Our excitement had been short-lived and she cried harder than I'd ever seen her cry. Ali, the transplant coordinator, talked her through it, assuring her that even though she wasn't a match, they'd find someone on the registry who was, and that I didn't need a transplant right away.

Thank you, Mr Orderly

The intense chemotherapy made me continually neutropenic so I had to stay in my isolation room to avoid exposure to germs. I craved the outdoors every day. I had never been locked up inside for so long. I was used to running and working outside and my whole childhood had been spent enjoying nature.

One day I was let out of my isolation room to attend an appointment for my eye.

Even though I was exhausted and an utter mess, I got so excited at the prospect of an outside excursion. It was a cold day. They warmed blankets and wrapped me up from head to toe in white. I wore a face mask to prevent any bugs getting to me. My head dangled to the left, eyelids drooping over tired eyes. No eyebrows, no hair on my head; all anyone could see of me was pinhole eyes in my flopping head.

The orderly took me to my appointment down a long corridor. As we were waiting for the elevator, I saw a young girl. I can only imagine how I must have looked to her: a skeleton wrapped in blankets. She was staring at my pinhole eyes. I slipped my hand out from the sheets and gave her a weak wave and a smile. I forgot that with the mask over my mouth she couldn't see my grin. She grabbed her Mum's arm and turned away in panic as if a monster was trying to grab her.

My head went down and I sobbed quietly. I was a fucking monster.

After the appointment, I wanted to be outside so bad. I asked the orderly to wheel me out there.

'No, I can't do that. It's against the rules.'

Fuck, I hated rules. I said, 'Man, just take me outside, who cares if you get me sick. Please, man, can you?'

'No, sorry, mate. Can't do it.'

I used the remnants of my energy to tell a lie and make my voice firm with it. 'Please take me outside. I only have a week left to live. Please, please.'

He sighed and said, 'Okay, mate, but you can't tell your nurses or your doctor.'

'I won't. Thank you!'

My excitement grew as the wheelchair approached the doors. When they opened, a great gust of wind flowed over my head, face, and through my mask. It was so fresh and pure, like silk on my skin. For the first time in 20 days I actually felt alive.

How good it was to see the leaves rustling and fighting in the wind. I wanted more. I wanted to embrace it all and take it with me so I pretended to grab the wind in my hand. I had never experienced nature so acutely before and it felt as if God Himself was touching me and saying, 'You will be okay'.

Life was blown back into me. I wanted to live for the wind and the sounds of the leaves gusting along the path and playing with such reckless abandon. I'd always felt the wind when I was running, warm and comforting on a mild day, but now I could *see* it with my eyes. The moment was short but it gave me the motivation I needed to go back in and fight for the life I loved.

I returned to my room with a smile. My focus was back. Thank you, Mr Orderly, from the bottom of my heart, for taking me outside. That short moment gave me the courage I needed. My fight became easier.

I had never really felt the wind until that day. I saw the wind and the wind saw me. We became good friends and I longed for its company every day.

I'd had a taste of all that was waiting for me. Life entered me again.

Ranui House

That one breath of fresh air sustained and inspired me to fight the constant fatigue, diarrhoea, vomiting and pain. Some days the exhaustion was overwhelming. Fatigue tormented me and I fought it hard. The simplest things took immense effort: getting up from bed and putting my clothes on. I'd struggle through the next minute, then the next hour. The prospect of facing the whole day all at once was just too daunting.

A month after the first chemo cycle my white blood cell count came back up and I moved out of isolation and into Ranui House, which Mum had told me was like a brand-new hotel. Ranui House was established by an incredible woman Allison Nicol, who became a great friend. Her son had leukaemia when he was a young boy. Allison recognised how families needed accommodation during long term treatments and she created a foundation – The Bone Marrow Cancer Trust. It truly is a 'home away from home'. Mum and Rachael had a two-bedroom self-contained unit where I could also stay. A short walk from my outpatient appointments – when I met Dr Peter Ganley to discuss where the cancer was at, the drugs I was taking, whether blood results meant I needed a transfusion – the House became my sanctuary, a home away from home. How grateful I was for a bed with warm, soft blankets where I could sleep in peace with no monitors, or nurses coming in. Every time I stayed there, a smile grew on my face and the pain of my situation disappeared for a while.

I never saw other patients while in isolation at the Unit. At Ranui House I met others receiving treatment for different types of cancers and it was good to share stories. I walked outside as much as I could, breathing in my newfound friends: the wind and the fresh air. I was appreciating the taste of coffee and the energy to laugh and to cry.

Most days I walked around the block or across the road to Hagley Park. I felt so blessed that this beautiful, green place was on my doorstep. Although walking was always a struggle against fatigue, the rewards were worth it.

Every day brought something new, things that had always been there and I'd never noticed, like the crunch of a passerby's footstep, a bird's soft tune, the wind's gentle hum in my ears. Small, precious things gave me such inner joy. I was so grateful to be able to sit and watch, to feel all that surrounded me, to be alive.

The cool winter air and the fresh wind fed my soul, fulfilled and inspired me. I looked up at the sky and watched the birds, envious of their high-flying freedom, not a care, embracing the wind with their flight.

Sometimes, in spite of the cold, I put my bare feet on the grass. It reminded me of running free as a kid, no worries and the whole day in front of me. If I fell, I picked myself up and ran on with the sun beating down, heard the laughter of the other kids all around, no rules, just fun. Out of the Unit, I rediscovered that forgotten child and laughed at all that had transpired over the last month. I hobbled around, weak and tired, but embracing my hard-won freedom with joy, a contented smile and open arms.

Daily visualisation and prayer helped. I pictured myself running, floating and playing in the wind. I wanted so much to understand life and death, the feelings I was having about my own mortality, and to make some sense of all I was experiencing. I didn't want to die, but I became aware of the possibility and unafraid at the thought of death. Dying was a part of life too, but this was not the way I wanted to die, not just yet.

Sometimes I wondered if life was about love, nothing more, nothing less. I started to feel my life from the heart, becoming sure of what I loved and the people in my life whom I loved.

My stay at Ranui House was short-lived and I was soon back in my wee room for another round of chemo, another battle. I was back in the cancer world. Deep in my heart, I held onto all that I loved.

It was always there.

Second cycle and say hello to Poley

I had lumbar punctures three times a week, injecting chemotherapy into my spinal cord. This was reduced to two per week after the first month, then until my treatment finished. I was thin and an ideal practice subject for the registrars because they could see my vertebrae. They often hit nerves that made my right or left leg spaz out of control. Each round of chemo was hard, with constant nausea and a lot of crying in the bathroom. Every day I woke up feeling like an old man.

My friends visited daily. I smiled during the brief time they were with me. I carried the frustration and pain inside – it was always there – and if I tried to put my feelings into words, they replied, 'Yeah, well, I bet it's tough, just stay positive, mate, and you'll be right.'

In my head I was shouting, Stay positive? Is that the best you can do? Fuck off then, let me be angry. Everything I had is gone and you're telling me I'll 'be right'?

When my visitors left, I was alone, dealing with the constant nightmare question of whether I'd live or die. The longer I was in isolation, the more negative the thoughts became. I hated being locked up.

One loyal friend was always there for me, never said anything, and was skinnier than me.

'Poley' was the stand and pole holding all of my medications. He was my life support. If my line got air in it or I rolled over in my sleep, Poley would beep and siren. I'd swear at him, tell him to fuck off, but he never did. He followed me everywhere like a bad smell. The bags of medication were attached to him, and then to my Hickman line. We were inseparable, Poley and I. He listened outside as I cried in the toilet, stood sentinel by my bed morning and night, responding to me with the constant clack of the machine he held. My mate Poley. I hated him but I loved him.

I finished the second cycle, got out again and started smoking. I snuck out of Ranui House to sit on a bench next to the canal and light up in the darkness of night, hoping no one would see me. I was caught between two extremes: loving and embracing the small joyous things, then at night when my head hit the pillow, wandering into a dungeon of hate and self-pity. Smoking helped take away the dark thoughts. I needed something, anything, and the cigarettes gave me a head spin. After seven cigarettes I thought, What the fuck am I doing? This shit causes what I have. And I had to laugh because the drugs they gave me worked far better at spinning my head anyway. My smoking days ended.

Looking back, I see that the smoking reflected my downward spiral. Cigarettes serve no purpose other than death, plain and simple.

Not talking

I can still see Mum's face when I was diagnosed at Greymouth Hospital. It had scared me more than the words, 'You have cancer.' I'd always been a mummy's boy and to see her face drop, and her eyes start to stream tears hurt so much. I thought, Did I do this to Mum? I'm causing her pain. I wanted to protect her and so I told her it would be okay. I told myself that too. I never wanted Mum and

Dad there when the doctors had news for me and I never gave my parents the full story. I was determined to get this done on my own. It was a burden I didn't let anyone else share.

This was a mistake. I needed to talk. Not asking for help meant locking myself away in the toilet or taking my anger out on Dad.

During her stays at Ranui House, Mum cooked food and brought it over to me. I had always known the importance of healthy food and having Mum so close, providing me with delicious alternatives to the hospital meals, was a blessing. Through my big window facing the park I could see her coming. And yet, watching Mum scared me because I believed I was hurting her. She always had a worried look that sometimes turned to terror. Was she scared *of* me, or *for* me?

I reassured her every day, saying, 'I'll be okay,' but I could never share my deepest feelings with her and I ached to do just that. I couldn't tell her about the traumatic and painful experiences I was having, the tears I cried almost daily. I suspect she knew. I tried to laugh, be upbeat and tough, saying I wanted this done and I'd finish it as I would a job at work so I could get on with the things I loved. This inability to talk eventually consumed me. My anger grew. I cried more. I lacked the strength to put my hand up and say, 'I need help.'

My friends came into my isolation room and talked about their relationships, fears and worries. I listened and made suggestions. They all wanted to help me too, and I appreciated the messages and the kind intention behind them, knowing they found it difficult to know what to say. But I never told them what was on my mind. I got sick of hearing the words, 'Stay positive', over and over. It was too hard to 'stay positive', have a 'positive outlook', and put up a 'positive fight' because being negative and letting frustrations out was part of the journey too.

I longed to say, 'Hey, instead of trying to find words to make me feel better, can you just say, "Hello"? Simple!' Advice or stories about other people's cancers were not helpful. Their journeys were not mine and hearing about someone who had endured a different cancer, or who had passed away, never made me feel better.

What I needed more than anything was a listening ear, some hearty laughter and a good cry over the hardship, with shared tears to wash away the pain.

With the wisdom of hindsight, I say to those suffering, 'Let the negativity out or it will eat you alive. Vent frustration, then carry on. Say thank you, show respect, treat everyone with a smile even if they don't understand.' But I wasn't there yet.

It'd be so easy to jump

They say that every journey has a low point, when you hit the dark, rock-bottom, where you make a decision to either give up and stay there, or start climbing out.

One evening, halfway through my treatment, I was staying with Mum and Rachael at Ranui House. They stepped out for a while and I was alone in the living room chair.

I wanted to die. All of the shit had to stop. I had completely lost the self I knew and had no idea now what life was about. It would be far easier to end it all.

My mind would not turn off. It kept telling me that I'd lost everything. No person would love me ever again. I'd never run or work again. I longed for my past, and Josh the 'fastest runner'. I anguished over the goals that had been snatched away when I was in the best shape of my life. I'd put in so many gruelling training hours, sacrificed so much to achieve that strength and fitness and here I was, weak, lost, confused and wanting to die.

The mental tirade did not stop. I was weak and pathetic, a burden to my family. It went on and on like an incessant, loud fire alarm I couldn't shut off. I was crying, grabbing my head with my hands and squeezing it tight, shouting, 'Shut the fuck up!'

I walked to the balcony and looked down. I'd always loved jumping off things, especially bridges and down into water, so leaping from the balcony seemed like a good way to end my life. I thought, Yes, I can do this. One jump and I'll be gone. Jump, Josh, jump. Just do it then all the pain will be over.

I put one leg over the railing. Then I looked back and saw Mum's cup of tea on the table. I saw her so clearly in my mind and knew with such clarity how devastated she would be. I could not leave her with tears for the rest of her life. I had to keep going for her. I loved my mum so much and could not take this way out. I had to go on.

Pure love embraced me in that moment. I had lost everything – my strength, my health, my happiness and nearly my mind– but love for my mother brought me back like a lightning bolt. My mum who nurtured me as a kid and was here caring for me now.

All the other people in my life popped into my head. I realised how much my brother, sister and dad loved me, and my friends Hamish and Ruth. I walked away from the balcony, back into the room, head down and crying hard.

That night I popped two sleeping pills and woke to start another day in the knowledge that I would never do that again. I accepted that it was okay to cry and be weak. And it was time to get real help. I summoned all of my strength to ask for it, because it was me, and only me that was responsible for my pain and suffering. No one else could walk the path for me. The load on my shoulders was far too heavy, so to be responsible I had to ask for help.

Canteen to the rescue. 'You're not using all your strength if you don't ask for help.'

Canteen is a wonderful charity supporting young people experiencing cancer. They hooked me up with psychologist David Garb. Together we talked deeply about life and death and he gave me valuable skills and tools to help deal with the pain and negative thoughts.

David said I could take ten minutes each day to cry, scream and say all the shit I wanted, then I was to go about my day in a positive manner. I kept to the regime, allowing myself only the allocated amount of time to let loose.

David taught me how to communicate and share my problems. I learned to speak about my feelings more openly, always coming back to how I would get through this, rather than being stuck in the torture of 'why me?' I knew my limited strength was far better spent learning more about my disease, thinking constructively and asking for help when I needed it.

David asked me to write 70 times a day for seven days, 'I, Josh Komen, love myself for the person I am.' Soon I felt my old self returning, and I grew stronger mentally. I wrote in my diary every day, expressing my feelings through words. If I was having a tough day, I'd manage only a handful of words, but on other days I wrote far more. The writing became an outlet and helped pass the time in my isolation room. It helped me get my thoughts in order and added reality to my dreams. I drew pictures. I saw myself running out on the Coast Road, smiling, happy and free. In my mind I was the Josh I so wanted to be. I trained myself to use a routine of visualisation, focusing every hour on the picture of a happy, strong and healthy Josh. I looked at the beautiful trees swaying in the wind, watched people going about their daily business, and saw the ducks, swimming, flying and eating in the park. I wanted to be like a duck, content and free to wander.

I began to plan the life that I wanted, jotting down ideas for adventures like becoming a skydiver and going to Everest Base Camp.

Passing the time in isolation

It was a lonely place, day after day, with only myself for company. Many of my thoughts revolved around death, life, pain, suffering, people and nature. I would chat to the nurses and friends would visit, but most of the time I was alone. I rarely watched TV or movies. I preferred to sit in my bed, watch the wind and the trees, write in my diary and listen to music, which I loved.

I watched the people go by, trying to read their minds and imagine what they were thinking.

I thought about my past and relived many hours, learning more and more about myself all the time. What had I done that was good? What should I have done? Why did I do or say this or that? Then my mind would launch onto a future track. How can we control the pain? Will I live or die, and if I live, what will I do?

I had endless hours to see myself from the inside out, to really say hello and get to know Josh Komen as a person. As I grew inside, I felt freer, less confined to the generally accepted way of living one's life. Slowly I was understanding that suffering was a part of life, everyone had their own problems and this was my problem. And if I could get through this problem, this pain I suffered, I would become stronger for it.

Sure, this world isn't fair, and life certainly isn't. We all face difficulties and challenges. Being by myself so much made me forget about things that used to have importance: the sex, drugs, alcohol, watching TV, obeying the system, trying to live up to the image the world expected. The many times I felt like a lost child, it was because I had forgotten my inner self, my soul, my breath of life.

I was a loner, but a curious one, wanting to feel and to understand what made me tick. The pain I endured had, in some inexplicable way, set me free to love fully and completely, with my heart and soul. Love was something that could never be taken from me. It would always be there inside, the only answer, burning brightly. It was up to me to decide how big the flame should grow.

When the pain came, I told myself it was a good thing because it meant I was alive. Pain was my friend, a sign of life. I laughed at it, cried with it, spat at it, embraced the stink of vomit because it all meant I was still alive and fighting. The climb up the hill got steeper and steeper. Reminding myself that everything will come to an end, like a race, or a day's work, meant I never let the hill grow too big and always kept the top in sight. When I reached the top – the end of this chemo, this treatment, this hospital stint – then I'd be back doing the things I loved with the comfort of walking down. This was my daily mental practice.

From time to time, I felt envious. My physical strength was gone and I couldn't do the simplest things that others did so effortlessly, nor could I do what I loved. Mental power became my strongest asset. I focused on reaching my goals. I had my friend the wind, my life, and my family. I wanted to live for them, find a girlfriend and fall in love.

The nurses were in my corner and I was grateful for their compassionate support and care. They were always upbeat, joking and laughing, and made such a difference in my day. They also saw my anger and tears.

After accepting that I needed to talk, I opened up to Nurse Mikayla. She had a great sense of humour and was a good listener. She called me Trouble because every shift something would happen: my blood pressure would drop or go up, or I'd spike a temperature.

Nurse Nic saved my life. I was having a bag of platelets infused. Platelets are clotting agents that keep you from bleeding out. It must have been a bad bag because I had an anaphylactic reaction to it. I felt this sense of impending doom and hit the buzzer three times as I struggled to breathe. Nic administered the adrenaline needed to bring me back.

I was in the Bone Marrow Unit for about four months in total. I had my fourth and final cycle of chemotherapy and managed well because my body was getting used to it. I was sleeping better, excited about getting out and had no plans to come back, even though Dr Peter said there was a high likelihood that my cancer would return so I needed to live and do whatever my head and heart desired.

I ignored the warning about relapse. This would never happen. I was getting out and would start rebuilding my worn-out body and mind.

Going home

My first night back home in Greymouth I cried and cried.

It was October 2011, still quite cold and wet in Greymouth and overcast, like my mind. What had just happened to me? The mind was flooded with thoughts.

I had spent the last seven months in and out of isolation, in immense pain, having been told I could die. Then just like that I was back home in one world – back where I had begun. What was the last seven months about? I felt like a lost soldier returning from war.

The cancer journey wasn't over just because I'd finished treatment. Despite the good strategies I'd been learning, now I felt lost, angry and full of self-pity. I was back living at home with Mum and Dad while my mates where adventuring around the world. I felt young at heart, old in body and mind. I began to wonder if being out was any better than the loneliness of my little room in the Unit.

All I'd known before illness was training, fitness and work. Now, I was weak, tired, unable to run. There was no returning to life as it had been before and I didn't know how to live this new one. I would have to become a new Josh.

I knew I'd grown as a person. I'd suffered so much pain. My thoughts had changed too and I worried that people would think me a freak. I kept to myself as I walked about outside with my head in the breeze, away from my isolation room.

I struggled to talk to people and couldn't relate to some. Most wanted to go for a beer. I didn't want to touch alcohol and the smell of it made me nauseous. There were people I trusted, and I came out a little, sharing my thoughts and feelings. I knew who would listen and not try to give me advice. I found companionship with two men in particular who hadn't experienced cancer but had gone through tough times: my neighbour John Olsen and good mate Wayne Dwyer. These two were trustworthy older men who listened, and when they spoke it was direct, with empathy and understanding. They knew I needed to get my strength back, appreciated my emotional connection to nature, and supported me.

I couldn't run so began walking to regain fitness. More than anything, I needed to put on weight so I ate a lot of good food. I went surfing that whole summer. The water gave me the solace I needed.

If there was no swell I'd still paddle out on my board and sit, saying thank you to God and marvelling at how beautiful my home town was, how generous everyone had been, fundraising for me when I was in hospital. The wind was always at my back, a constant and reassuring presence. I sat on the ocean and thought about where I had been, who I had become, and what to do with my future.

My body gained strength, my hair grew back, my stamina increased and the fatigue lessened.

Being so fit before cancer helped. Within two months I was surfing the Cobden break, walking the Elizabeth Point track and a few hills around town, and enjoying my old stomping ground out on the Coast Road.

Fulfilling dreams: Nepal

When they drink too much, take too many drugs, smoke cigarettes or eat shit food and not exercise, people say to me, 'You might as well die of something.'

Wrong choice of words. I prefer, 'Choose to live for something,' and find whatever it is that fulfills, emotionally and physically. Choose good health because it offers a fighting chance of beating a life-threatening illness.

My recovery was aided by my running background, an active, healthy lifestyle, and having a purpose. My body came back quicker than I expected and I started making plans to fulfil dreams.

Ben called one day and asked if I wanted to go to Everest Base Camp. The dream of being there had sustained me during all the months of pain and the offer excited me. I had some doubts, though. Would I be strong enough to manage the trip? Would I get sick in Nepal?

My mind drew 'yes' then 'no' out of a hat at least ten times a day until one afternoon out in the surf, I said, 'Yeah, fuck it, you gotta do it, man.' Slapping the water hard as the sun hit my face, I let out a wolf cry of pure delight. Yes, I would travel to Nepal. Going with

Ben, one of my best childhood mates, made it even more special.

Within five months of discharge from hospital, my body was thriving. I felt like a kid again. I was free. No needles, no chemo, blood or platelet transfusions, just good pain as I pushed my body, walking on the hills again, slow and steady, nothing rushed. My recovery was well paced and I was tuned in to what I could handle.

I was going to Nepal. All my earlier fears seemed surreal and pointless. I was on my way with a backpack and a smile no man could take from me. Nepal would be one of the best experiences of my life.

When I walked out of the Kathmandu airport hundreds of men were yelling, 'Come, taxi for you, taxi for you!' The smell was intense, like weeds burning in a paddock. It was like being at a concert, right in front of the stage, overwhelmed by the buzz of the crowd. Sweat and heat together made a tiny fire inside me and soon I was dripping. As my inner fire grew, so did my excitement at being as far from the Bone Marrow Unit as I could possibly get. This was adventure, life. The pain had been worth the suffering to experience this overwhelming moment of the crazy taxi men yelling and screaming at me.

I found my man, and said with a grin, 'Let's go!' Freedom, pure freedom. No rules, no chemo, no pain, just me, my backpack and a mad tuk-tuk driver. As we drove to my hostel, my head swivelled, trying to take in all of the sights – litter everywhere, so many people walking in the mud, the dirt road full of big potholes. I felt fortunate to have been treated for cancer in New Zealand. There seemed to be hundreds of people sleeping on the street or in their tuk-tuks and it seemed unlikely they would receive adequate health care for serious illness. My worries and my life seemed insignificant compared to the daily realities for these Nepalese people.

It was then I realised I was grateful to suffer in such comfortable conditions – those people had nothing – yet in my hospital room I had a shower and a warm bed. I closed my eyes and thanked God that I had suffered in comfortable surroundings.

Ben flew in the next day. We were both so excited about our

adventure and couldn't get the smiles off our faces. With the help of local people, one in particular whom we tipped generously, we obtained our mountain permit, the supplies we needed and our airline tickets to Lukla.

They say Lukla is one of the world's most dangerous airports. It has an elevation of 2,860 metres, the landing strip is short and ends on the edge of a cliff. The flight in was amazing. The mountains came alive: huge, the biggest in the world, towering over our little plane.

I was blown away, too, by the pure love of the Nepalese and I still hold their smiles in my heart. The Western world would say, 'These people have nothing,' but they had happiness and love for themselves and family. It was so simple. From the start, I enjoyed talking to people and listening to their stories. They spoke so politely and shared so openly. It wasn't just the mountains that where big. The Sherpas and Nepalese had huge hearts, the mountains reflecting their strong determination.

The trek to Base Camp

The trek was tough. We carried our own backpacks. Our guide Mingma wore a smile, jeans, a light jacket and old shoes and patiently answered all of our questions about the area and the Sherpa people. I looked in awe at the mountains all around, so beautiful, scary, inviting and majestic.

The altitude took its toll on me and one night I became unwell. My body needed food and deep sleep. I visualised my goal of getting to Base Camp with Ben, carrying my own pack the whole way. The following day I was groggy but better. The trek to the next village was shorter, and we went slowly. Ben encouraged me to continue, one step at a time. We made it and decided to stay two nights to get used to the altitude and thin air. Then we were on our way again to Everest Base Camp.

Strength was put into perspective for me when I saw an old man with a freezer. He was carrying it to the next village, up the steep trail, a rope bound around his head and the freezer hanging off his back. His head was down, no doubt his quad muscles were burning, and he walked in sandals. When I worked on the lines out of Greymouth we had so much gear to make the job easier. Here they had nothing but pure strength and determination.

Slowly but surely it took us just over one week to make our way to Base Camp. Both Ben and I came around an open bend on the trail and there was Mt Everest, right in front of us. To see the mountain had been my dream and I was living it, grateful to be there, witnessing such beauty and experiencing real adventure.

I hugged Ben when we reached Base Camp. It had been a struggle. I revelled in the satisfaction of fulfilling a dream, returning from the brink of death to life and freedom.

The suffering all seemed worth it. I felt sheer gratitude, being in one of the most beautiful places on earth. I held my hands high, took in my surroundings and thanked God for what I had achieved, where I was, who I was with, and most of all, for my life.

I had achieved my goal, a life's dream, and now I knew that if I focused my mind on something, I could turn more of my dreams into realities.

The next morning Ben and I trekked up a mountain called Mt Kala Patthar. There we watched the sun rise over Mt Everest, a joyous moment. We were 18,1921 feet above sea level and I felt as if I could touch the mountain itself. This was a small perfect moment in life that few people experience. I closed my eyes and savoured this moment, acknowledging how good life can be when you persevere through pain.

Coming back down I felt sick. The delight of achievement was knocked back to the all-too-familiar 'one step at a time', telling myself to just keep walking. I had severe vomiting and diarrhea and had to get down so I could receive some medication.

We hiked from Base Camp to Namche Bazaar and on to Lukla Airport. Much was downhill but the uphill stretches were tough. I couldn't eat, and drank only small quantities of water. I pushed and pushed, focused on my steps, smiling in spite of it all. I was always telling myself: 'Josh you can get there, then you can sleep and they will sort you out. Just get there and the reward will be so satisfying.'

The boys I'd worked with before I had cancer always said, 'If you start it, you finish it,' so when Ben offered to take my pack I fought him off, saying, 'Fuck off, man! I start with my pack, I finish with my pack.' I confused him. He didn't understand my stubbornness. I started the trek with that pack and was going to finish it. I'd ask for help if I needed it. It was a battle, but the pain was nothing compared to the agony I had lived through during the months in Christchurch Hospital. I dug deep and finished the job.

I was so relieved when we staggered in to Lukla. Ben and I had a nice warm drink, a light dinner, and a deep sleep. I flew out to Kathmandu with a bag full of shitty undies and a contented smile on my face. I went to the doctor, got some pills and within 48 hours was eating like a horse again.

Nothing came easy but the pain was worth the reward. I had been given a prize no person could ever award me. The trek had made me more aware of myself as a person, and of what I could and couldn't do. I understood my limits and achieved what I needed to. It may not have been the top of Mt Everest, but Base Camp had been my own personal summit.

Thank you, Ben, for an experience I'll never forget and I apologise for nearly punching you when you were just trying to help.

Thailand

After the Base Camp adventure, we flew to Thailand for some R & R and found an island to just hang out on and relax. I took to island life right away: delicious food, gorgeous beaches, swimming and diving. It was the perfect place to recover. I'd attained my PADI license to dive in Greymouth before I left, so enjoyed the clear, blue water, floating around with the marine life as often as I could. Every evening I'd lie on the beach and listen to the crash of the ocean onto the shore. I laughed aloud over how good life was, as far from my isolation room as I could possibly be. I knew I had to give running another shot, come back stronger and faster than ever before.

Ben left after a week and I decided to remain in South East Asia. I had enrolled for the New Zealand Skydiving Diploma course in Methven, starting July 2012, ten weeks away. I wanted to make the most of the time. I appreciated life, my body was strong and I had forgotten about cancer. I backpacked through Thailand, crossed the border into Laos, slept some nights in Laotian jungle tree huts in the middle of nowhere, and met a cool group of people to travel with.

Meeting Clara

I first saw Clara in a long boat heading down the Mekong River. She was sitting on one side of the boat by herself. I sat on the opposite side and we were both admiring the view. I was taking in everything: the people, scenery, smells, the feel of the wind, while most others on board were either drinking or drunk.

Clara stood out. She wore a singlet in my favourite bright green. Her bare feet dangled comfortably, her hair played with the light breeze dancing through the boat. I watched carefully as her big, beautiful, curious eyes took in the new terrain. She held her head out, face to the wind, so the cool air could flow through her hair. Her face reflected the delight she got from doing such a simple thing. I wanted to talk to her. I knew she was different, and special.

We did talk. I told her about myself and she said her home was a small town in Germany called Schloss Hamborn, a peaceful organic village. Clara came from a loving family and was very open-minded about the world. At just 20, she had recently hitch-hiked around New Zealand by herself. I was impressed. We enjoyed each other's company and shared conversation about our lives and experiences.

On that same boat trip, I met other like-minded people who became my friends and travelling companions. There were Sanne and Dan from the USA, Bas and AJ from Holland, Alberto from Italy, Clara and her friend Lea. We traveled through Laos together, riding on scooters along rugged roads, having adventures and enjoying each other.

After our trip through Laos, Dan and I decided to hitch-hike through the northern part of Cambodia. We were both keen to get off the beaten track and see the real countryside and people, the parts the tourists never went to. We planned to meet up with the group again in Siem Reap to visit Angkor Watt.

We picked up a basic map at a local market. It unfolded to the size of a door, looked like it had been drawn by children, and had no real detail. Undaunted, we set off armed with our giant kids' map, small backpacks and curiosity. Our first ride was in a four-wheel drive. The driver was in charge of constructing a new road so we went with him to the end of that, then walked about ten minutes to the nearest small village. We had no idea what town we were in, where to stay or find food, so we wandered into a park full of young children playing soccer. The game was crazy with about 50 kids chasing the ball. We asked if we could join and they were all so happy for us to play. It was tough, running around and trying to keep up with these kids! Their rules were different so Dan and I ended up just chasing the ball as the kids laughed with delight. After the game, a young boy asked if we would like to visit his school. 'Of course!' we said.

So off we went. The sole teacher wanted us to teach the class some English. I have never seen such enthusiasm and curiosity in school kids before. The classroom was just four walls – not colourful posters or pictures – and about 20 pupils with straight backs, hunger for learning on their faces, and no equipment besides pieces of paper and pencils. Forget the whiteboards and computers of a New Zealand classroom. These children were keen to learn, work hard and make a better life for themselves. They touched my heart. They had such smiles, were inquisitive and full of excitement. I talked about my home country New Zealand, and when I asked them what they would like to be when they were older, 90 percent replied, 'Doctor!' These children had little but wanted so much from life, approaching their goals with energy and patience.

Dan and I had a meal with the principal at a local eatery, where we ate with our hands. He told us that the children don't have much but they have each other and strong family bonds.

As we ate he told us about an old temple that was being held by the Cambodian army. Apparently, people had died there. Of course, our ears pricked up and we decided to visit. The principal kindly found us a place to stay for the night and the next morning we hitched a ride on a tractor with an old man delivering water to the rural houses along the beaten-down road. Dan and I sat on the trailer with the water containers and helped with the deliveries, saving him time and effort getting off and on. Few words were spoken. He smiled all the time and gave us the universal thumbs-up in appreciation of our efforts.

Our next ride was with two boys on a scooter. There we were, four of us with our backpacks, crammed on the scooter like monkeys. We rode 20 km with the boys until they said the ride would become too dangerous for all of us, so we hopped off and started walking down the dusty dirt road on a hot humid day with our thumbs out.

Eventually a young family in a small car took us another 30 km along the rugged road, dodging potholes all the way. One of the young kids in the car stared at us with curiosity. The father driving could see his son in the rear vison mirror. He chuckled and said, 'First time my son see white man.' We all laughed then and I said hello to the small boy who was very shy.

An ambulance picked us up next, and took us to the Cambodian army training centre. We had coffee with the soldiers and stayed the night in a small town that was a 25 km ride away from the temple.

Early the next morning we rented scooters and headed out. As we'd been informed, the Cambodian army was holding the area. I had my camera and said we were working for National Geographic so they let us through. Whether they believed us was another story – I think it helped our bid for entry that we handed over some American dollars – but we passed the army guard and reached the temple, high on a ridge. Dan and I had the whole place to ourselves and we climbed all over the open temple ruins like kids in a castle or a huge abandoned playground.

We waited for the sunset. The whole valley lit up in sparkling gold, an incredible show just for the two of us. It paid to venture off the beaten path, accept random rides, meet the real people of the country, and experience one of the most glorious sunsets I have ever seen.

Seeking Pol Pot

Our next mission was to get to the Cambodian dictator Pol Pot's hideout. Pol Pot led the notorious Khmer Rouge, the regime responsible for the Cambodian genocide between 1975 and 1979 of between 1.5 and 3 million people. We arrived at the town nearest to the hideout and a young boy approached us. 'What are you doing? People are asking questions.' We explained that we were looking for Pol Pot's hideout and the boy said he would take us there for 50 USD. We gave him the money and away we went, three of us on his scooter through dense, muddy jungle terrain.

We travelled for about 15 km, through jungle creeks and mud. Forget the all-terrain vehicles; this was Cambodian scooter 4WD driving. Further into the jungle we came across small huts full of men and women, cautious and wondering what we were up to. Our young friend told them politely and they said we could carry on only if we stopped and drank some home-made spirits with them. With some hesitation we drank and continued our journey.

We came across the hideout, all but hidden amongst tall weeds and the trees that soar above it. The underground bunker was full of water with a lookout hole affording a view of the valley below. Not much to see, but we were satisfied. We left, stopped for another drink with the men in the hut, then bounced back through creeks and mud to where we'd started.

What an experience. Dan and I laughed about what we'd just done and decided to head on to Siem Reap to tell Clara and the others about our adventure.

Happy and content, we met up with the crew, bragging to everyone about our journey and making them jealous.

Falling in love with Clara

Clara and I decided to leave the group and travel together. Biking through Angkor Watt, holding onto the tuk-tuk to get a fast tow, was such a thrill. Clara and I fell in love. I was so happy to be sharing my life with someone special. Cancer seemed far away.

Singapore was the final stop on our journey together. That last night, we went to one of the tallest buildings in the city, the Marina Bay Sands Hotel. A long infinity pool stretches across the front of three buildings and the view of the city is second to none. There was a $20 fee just to ride up, so we snuck past the guard, got in the elevator, rode the 57 levels up to the top, got a drink, left without paying, took the elevator back down and ran barefoot around the city, no cares in the world.

Clara and I had connected. She had a strong belief in herself and others, and understood my past. We had deep talks about life and what we both wanted, finding so much common ground, and there were tears when we parted. I was returning to New Zealand for skydiving school, and Clara to her home in Germany. We decided to leave our relationship open, see how much we would miss each other and, if it became unbearable, I would fly to Germany in a few months' time to see her. I loved this girl. We hugged and cried and acknowledged the special time we had spent together.

Skydiving

New Zealand is the only country in the world offering a seven-month diploma course in commercial skydiving and I was about to fulfill another dream. I got hooked at 19 on my first tandem skydive at Fox Glacier with Hamish and his partner Amy. The course was in Methven, near the Mt Hutt ski field, and I was so bloody excited about this opportunity to skydive full-time. I hoped the training would also prepare me for BASE jumping. I started the midwinter course in July 2012 and couldn't wait to take my first jump. Our coach and teacher was Gary Byer, a former world champion skydiver and one of the best instructors in the world. He had just taken up the role at the New Zealand Skydiving School, so our class was fortunate to have one of the very best teaching us how to jump safely out of planes.

On the very first day Gary said, 'Gentlemen, I'm about to change your life.' As I'd already been through a life-changing experience, I wondered how skydiving could possibly change it further. How naive I was; how could skydiving be anything but life-changing? Jumping out of a plane is not natural behaviour for a human being.

Gary was passionate and intense. He knew how to train and work hard, and have fun, and the course was everything I hoped it would be. I made lifelong friends and had the time of my life. The five other men on the course were Iohann from Brazil, Jarrod from Canada, Harley from Christchurch, Jason from Ashburton and Pariri from the North Island. We were training for AFF (Advanced Free Fall), learning the basics for solo jumping.

The first time up, my nerves were jangling and the adrenaline was flooding through me. I was about to jump out of a plane. My instructors Darren, Mason, Marika and Brent were all encouraging and calm. Brent fell asleep going up and all I could think was, 'Shit, I'm about to jump out of a plane and this dude is asleep! Does he even care?' But this was the skydive way, relaxed and calm about doing the extreme, controlling the mind.

It was time to jump with Mason and Brent. They held me side by side to ensure my body was positioned correctly, and we jumped. I don't remember much of that moment because the adrenaline had taken over. I opened my chute. The first sensation was a flood of relief that it had worked and then there I was, all alone, sitting in my harness with my chute floating above me and the earth below my feet.

This was the moment I became a skydiver: in the sky like a bird, alone in a vast world I'd only ever seen from below. I felt the rush of my good mate the wind, wrapping around me like a soft blanket. I smiled and cried with utter joy. I had never felt such freedom. How could this be so good? It was better than any drug I'd ever taken. Pure freedom. Addictive. I was hooked.

I landed well, shouting with joy and passion, 'Fuck yes! I just jumped out of a fucking plane!' I was so proud because I had fulfilled another of my childhood dreams and I was ready for more.

We worked on our jumps every day, learning how to fly our bodies in the wind. I'd wake up each morning, run the 15 km to the drop zone, have a cold shower (there was no hot water), then jump all day. The boys and I became great mates. Darren offered Harley and me accommodation in his shed and we gladly moved in. I was living the dream, so grateful to be where I was, doing what I loved, experiencing such freedom with the sky all to myself and the wind filling my body with pure life.

I Skyped Clara often, and we shared our days, feelings and adventures. I was content. I had an amazing girl in my life, was jumping out of planes and playing in the wind, having and doing everything I'd dreamed of.

One day Gary and I were talking and I told him about the cancer. He showed such empathy and understanding. We talked about running, and about being so competitive we lose sight of the enjoyment of our sport by trying too hard and caring too much. I realised I had cared too much about my performance, my times and results. I couldn't accept the not-so-good ones.

Sometimes I had lost sight of why I was running: for the freedom within, the pure enjoyment of pushing and feeling my heart beat through me, running in the rain, wind, sun, one foot after another, and the sheer joy of a beautiful view from the top of a hill. Sure, I wanted to win and represent my country but it wasn't all about winning.

When I was skydiving, whether it was a good or a bad jump, I was nevertheless leaping out of a plane, taking in breathtaking views of the snow-covered Southern Alps, and landing safely on the ground.

Feeling close to God

I never really believed in God growing up, but cancer had changed me. I felt life around me now. I respected everyone's beliefs and views. I often felt there was more to this life than I had or knew. It seemed as if someone was watching me, looking after me, moulding me into a better person.

Life became simple. Running, skydiving, whatever it was, I'd always wanted to be the best and find out as much as I could. Now I was learning a bigger lesson: to pause, see the big picture, and let in the love and enjoyment that comes from following your passion.

It was also about the people I was meeting on my journey: like-minded and extraordinary men and women I could relate to and share beautiful moments with, whether it be skydiving or accomplishing a tough training session together. It seemed that life was a path already mapped out and the people I met were the supporters clapping and encouraging me along the way.

I felt lucky to be alive. Instead of worrying about being the best, I came to care more about doing the best I could, not getting hung up when others made better jumps than me or flew a more bad-ass canopy. I distilled my awareness down to the simple action of doing what I loved, embracing the nature around me and the freedom I felt within.

I felt close to God when I was jumping, like I was in heaven. I thanked Him for the joy I felt in my heart when I was in the sky, something no one could take from me. I was in love with life and the person I was, growing every day, having fun and being a kid. When the door of the plane opened, a huge gush of wind flooded the cabin. My old friend welcomed me with a big hug every time. I couldn't wait for the plane to reach 12,000 feet, for the door to open so I could jump out and fly around with my mates, then spiral down beneath the parachute.

I met one of my best mates at skydiving school: Matt Walker. We spent a lot of time together and had so many common interests that his partner Millie said, 'If you were both gay you'd be a couple.' Matt and I had each lost a friend at a young age and we talked a great deal about life and death. Matt was keen on BASE jumping too (an acronym for places you can jump from: building, antenna, span, earth [cliff]) so on our days off we went to Christchurch gymnastics school to practise our gymnastics, backflips and front flips, in anticipation of doing a BASE-jumping course in the USA.

I'd been reading Lance Armstrong's book, *It's Not About the Bike*. His story of getting back on his feet after cancer gave me the motivation to run again. On the weekends I met up with my former mentor Don Grieg. He'd designed a rebuilding programme for me and I couldn't believe how quickly my body adapted to the training. After two months with Don, I was running five kilometres in 16 minutes, and taking on 25 kilometres each Sunday. I was doing so well I wondered if something in the chemo had changed my blood chemistry or homeostasis (the process to maintain a stable biological function), making me faster and stronger than ever before. I felt good and my fitness returned after more than a year and a half without training. If Lance could come back and win the Tour de France seven times then I could fulfill my dream of running for New Zealand.

In spite of his eventual exposure as a drug cheat, I respected Lance Armstrong for getting back on the bike. It takes a lot of effort to do what you love again after cancer has taken so much away. I was disappointed that he lied so blatantly to the cancer patients he inspired with his story, so I wrote him a letter saying that I admired him for getting back on his bike again, but that I hadn't liked being deceived by his lies.

Visiting Clara in Germany

The skydive course was government accredited so we had a two-week break over the October school holidays. Clara and I were missing each other so I took the opportunity to fly to Germany, meet her family and see the real Clara at home. I wondered if I was making a rash decision, and her parents did too, but if I felt something deeply

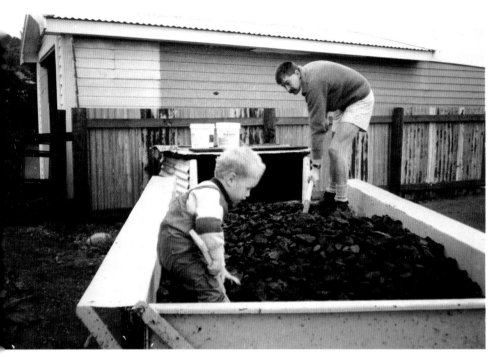

ABOVE: Shovelling coal with Dad — my father instilled a hard work ethic into me at a young age. Thanks, Dad. BELOW LEFT: Helping with the lambs at Grandad's farm in Whataroa. BELOW RIGHT: Running for Grey Main school at a young age — getting the win.

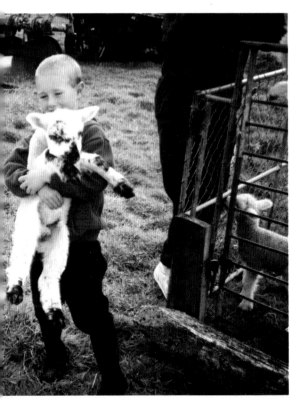

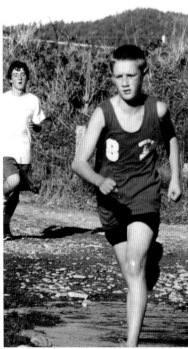

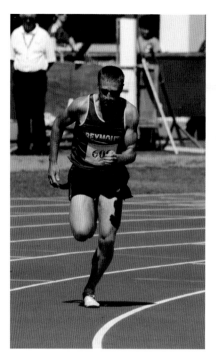 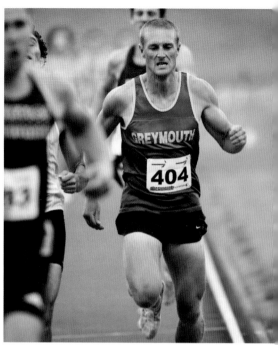

ABOVE LEFT: Off to a fast start. ABOVE RIGHT: Always proud to represent my hometown Greymouth. BELOW: Second place in my first Senior Men's New Zealand Championship 20 years old – a proud moment in my life.

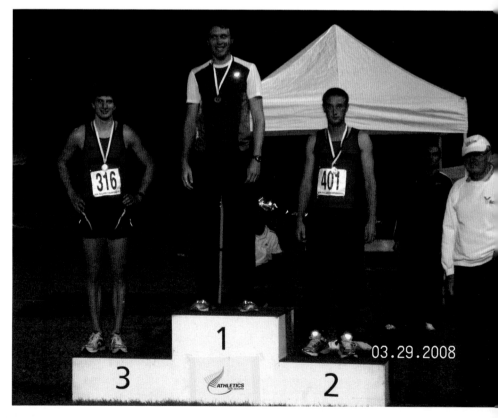

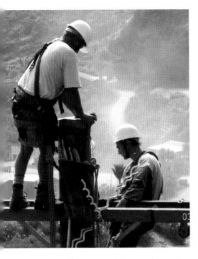
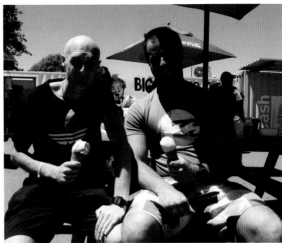

ABOVE LEFT: Ferny and I running wire with the helicopter. I loved these jobs. ABOVE RIGHT: My good mate, Hamish, he was always there to talk. BELOW: Me and my family: Rach, Mum, Dad and Jake — one month before I was diagnosed. You wouldn't even know I was sick.

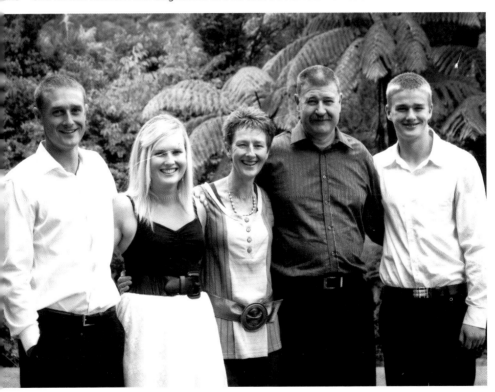

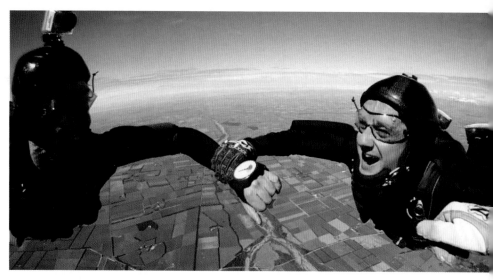

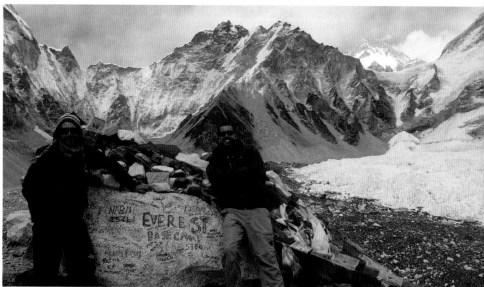

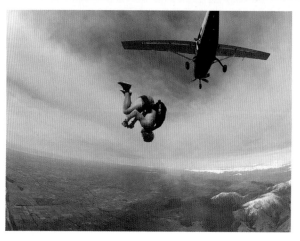

TOP: My good friend Iohann and I link up for a jump – the smile says it all.

ABOVE: Ben and I are proud to have achieved our childhood dream – Mt Everest Basecamp.

LEFT: On your 100th skydive it's tradition to jump in your underwear, hence the name 'undihundy'.

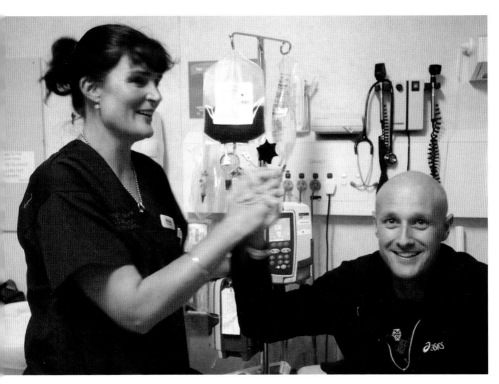

ABOVE: Transplant time – the bag in the background contains the stem cells that saved my life. With Nurse Mikayla. BELOW: My time in ICU – they say a picture paints a thousand words.

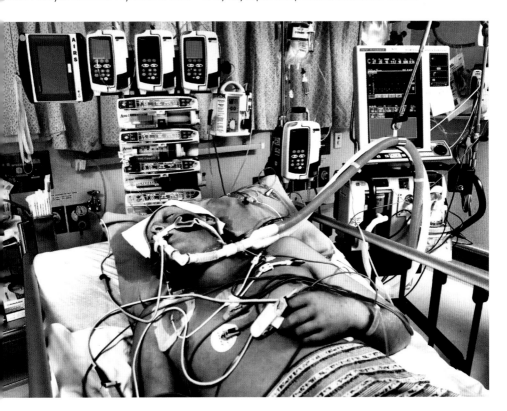

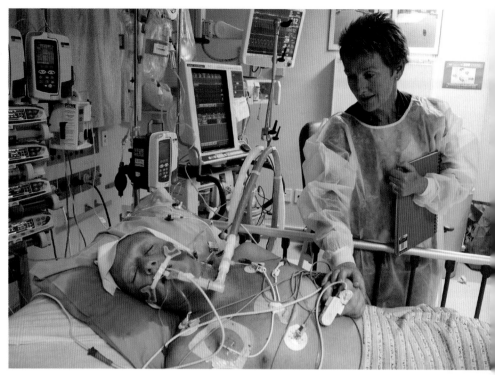

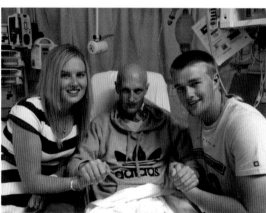

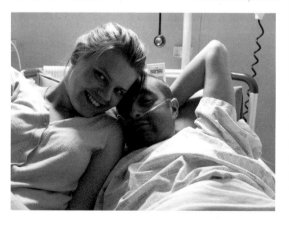

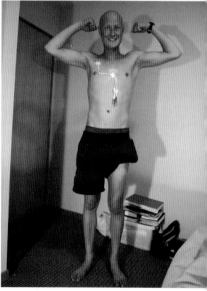

TOP: My strong mum never left my side.

ABOVE: Chemo can destroy the body and turn you in to an alien.

LEFT: My sister and brother, always there for me.

BOTTOM LEFT: Clara helped me a lot through my transplant.

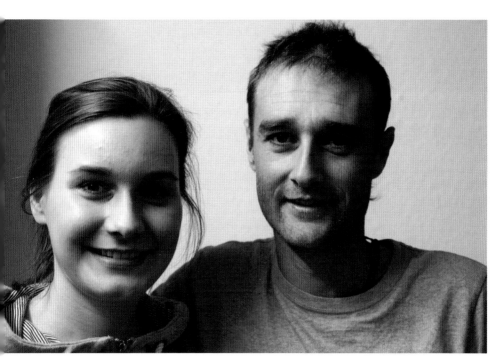

ABOVE: Not many transplant recipients get to meet their donor. It was an absolute privilege to meet Hannah, the girl who saved my life. I'm forever grateful, thank you. BELOW: The boys at 5th Element Wellness. From left: Mark, myself, Dave and Anthony. These three legends helped me a lot in Melbourne.

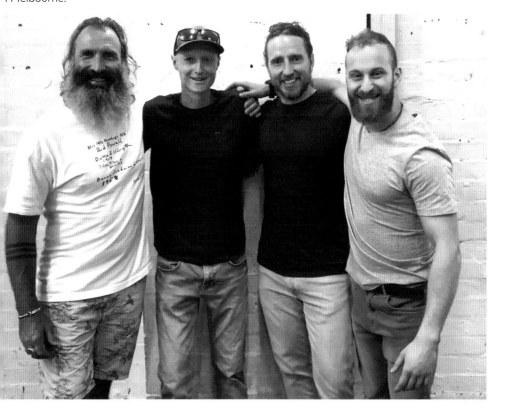

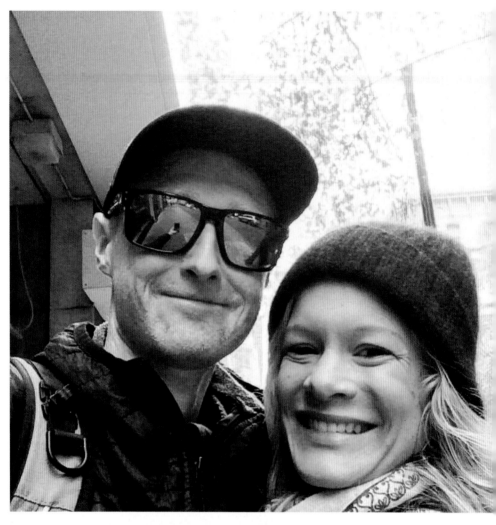

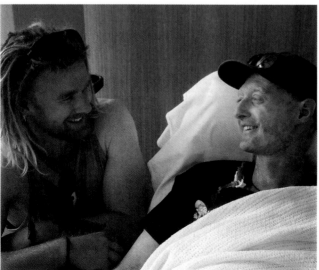

ABOVE: Sibille and I.
I'm definitely punching above my weight. Meeting Sibille gave me purpose through my pain. I love this girl!

LEFT: My great mate Jake, helping his brother where he can.

I went with it 100 percent. I loved Clara. My cancer had made me embrace everything and take every opportunity. I didn't want to die with any regrets.

I managed the long flight well. Seeing Clara again brought tears to my eyes and we reconnected in each other's arms, so happy to be together. Her family were loving and open. Her town of Schloss Hamborn was beautiful and I fell in love with the place. It was so picturesque with its cobbled streets and architecture, it was like living on a movie set. Deep orange and yellow-brown leaves lay scattered on the ground and the autumn air was fresh and cool, as it was in New Zealand. I could see myself living in this wee village. I felt no stress, no worries. The narrow streets and paths took me into a fairytale world, like stepping back in time. Leaves rained from swaying trees and crunched under my feet as I walked along.

Clara's parents, Sabine and Klaus, made me feel welcome. We talked about life, about my dreams and journey so far, and they accepted me into the family. Clara and I were officially a couple. I met Clara's older sister Elizabeth. She had a young son Noah with her partner Lukas. We all made a warm connection.

Clara and I spent a night in Berlin, a bustling city with so much going on. We saw the incredible Berlin wall. I met Clara's brother Jan who was a big strong lad but so friendly kind and welcoming. At the empty Berlin Olympic stadium, where New Zealand's own Jack Lovelock won the 1500 m gold medal in 1932, I managed to jump over the moat that kept the crowd off the track and run a lap. Afterwards, I jumped back over the moat just as a guard came over to kick me out. I was happy, though. I'd done my lap, pretending to be Lovelock.

My keen interest in World War II history meant that one night in Berlin wasn't enough. I left wanting more.

The day I left for home, Klaus drove me to the train station. We hugged and said our goodbyes. Klaus started to walk away, then he turned back and put his hands on my shoulders, looking deeply into my eyes. 'Stay alive,' he said. It was a strange way to say goodbye and I was taken aback. Was he concerned because I jumped out of planes, or did he think I would get sick again?

I knew that Clara's family often spoke with more meaning behind their words, and Klaus's words stayed with me. I wondered all the way home about what he had meant.

Happiness

Back at skydiving school, I felt no sadness, only enjoyment every single day of where I was and who I was with. I thanked God and acknowledged myself and my body with kindness and gratitude. It was great to be back, jumping with the beautiful Southern Alps as backdrop, and catching up with my new best mates Matt, Iohann and Wayne Holmes. Clara and I had decided she would come to New Zealand the following year, February 2013. I was excited about my future.

I washed dishes part-time in a local pub to help cover my course costs. I no longer drank alcohol, ate well, and there was never a dull moment hanging out with skydivers, a unique bunch of dudes. The members of my skydiving family came from a range of places and backgrounds, but we were united by our desire to learn and have fun. No one complained, everyone there was embracing life and all it could bring. We shared a profound love and respect for each other. Time passed quickly. My skills in the sky improved every day, and my running was consistent and strong.

At the start of November 2012 I noticed a scab on my arm. It wasn't healing. Matt and I continued our gymnastics and we were learning to do back flips. At one session, I tore a ligament in my knee and chipped a bone in my ankle. This injury didn't heal either and I was feeling tired. I took a few days off jumping.

Days of limping turned to weeks and then I noticed little purple spots appearing on my wrist. I remembered the poor healing and the spots from the first time. I allowed no emotion and carried on as normal. I told myself I didn't have cancer.

Deep down I knew that I did.

I didn't tell my schoolmates. I decided to wait until after my scheduled follow-up appointment with Dr Ganly, ten days away on 7 December. I wanted to jump as much as I could before seeing Dr Ganly and hearing him tell me the worst. I was like a kid in the playground, not coming in until Mum and Dad yelled so loudly that I had to. I managed a few more jumps even though I found them exhausting. My sweats came back and I was a dripping mess. After one jump, my mate Jack Par asked if I'd landed in the river. I laughed and said, 'Yeah, I wish!' knowing that would be far better than the real reason.

Stubborn Josh was back. I didn't want to accept that cancer had returned so I kept on jumping. I made a jump with a mate Ivan. Our plan was for a two-way belly jump, trying to do as many points (touching together) as possible: spinning and manoeuvring then coming back together. Jumping from 18,000 feet would give us more time falling and therefore more points. Climbing to that height meant we needed oxygen supplementation before we jumped. I felt dizzy and light-headed as soon as I took my oxygen mask off to open the door. I jumped and saw two Ivans, then three, then four. Holy shit, I was hypoxic, not getting enough oxygen to my organs. I slowly came to when I reached 8,000 feet, pulled my chute as soon as I could at 6,000 and landed safely, but dazed and confused. Ivan laughed and said, 'What the fuck were you doing up there, bro?'

'I don't know,' I said, foggy and stunned.

I was sick. I took a few sick days, struggling through the week before my appointment with Dr Ganly. This couldn't be happening, not again. I was content, the happiest I'd ever been. My fitness had been returning, I was enjoying my course, I'd made amazing new friends and I loved Clara so much.

On some level I was accepting because I knew, deep down, that the cancer could return. The doctors had told me this. I was glad that I'd followed my dreams, made it to Base Camp, travelled and had adventures, and learned to skydive. I was grateful for the time I'd been given to achieve all this. If I died this time, I'd have few regrets.

But I didn't want to go just yet.

PART THREE
CANCER AGAIN

God Grant me the serenity
to accept the things I cannot
change, courage to change
the things I can, and wisdom
to know the difference.

— IRISH PROVERB

IT WAS 21 November 2012, and here I was back again, back to the place I dreaded so much. My appointment with Dr Ganly in Christchurch confirmed that the cancer was back. Even though I knew, it was hard to hear him say the words. I sat on the seat in his office with tears running down my face, accepting but deeply disappointed. I was taken to a private office where I made the phone calls I dreaded. I heard the agony in the voices of my family, their cries and breakdowns into tears. This hurt me more than the news itself.

Mum and I cried together over the phone, but she was stronger than I thought. She'd had an inkling something was wrong because of my time off skydiving. I asked her to tell Dad and Rachael. My brother Jacob was away on his linesman apprenticeship course at the time. Then I asked, 'Would you, Dad and Rachael come and do a skydive in Methven with me before I start treatment?'

After hanging up from Mum I called my Aunty Rosie who was the clinical nurse specialist in the Orthopedics department at Christchurch Hospital. She was my 'Christchurch Mum', always there for me, providing good food, love, and a place to stay. She came running over and was the first person I hugged.

Then I had to tell Clara. It was the early hours of the morning in Germany and she was fast asleep. I broke the news and her cries over the phone cut me deep. I hate cancer for the pain and fear it brings to those I love. 'I'm coming over,' she said.

I went back to Methven, to tell Gary first. Gary had helped me so much, instilling better values into me, changing my thinking pattern, and best of all, he always challenged me. I grew so much at skydiving school with my new family. Gary had taught me not to care so much, to lighten up, have fun and enjoy what I did every day. Gary told us to work hard, achieve our goals and inner dreams, but also to stop and enjoy the scenery and be good, respectful, fun-loving people, not too hung-up on the small stuff. We were all on the same page with that.

I knocked on his door and he knew something was wrong without me saying anything. He grabbed my shoulders, we looked into each other's eyes and cried. My time at the school had ended.

I had to tell everyone on my course. They were shocked, horrified, and cried more than I did. Iohann, Matt, Wayne and my shed-mate Harley were devastated. My new brothers with whom I'd had so much fun in the sky. I had to leave them.

The big jump

Mum, Dad and Rachael agreed to do a tandem jump with me while I filmed them. My mum was so brave. Never in my life would I have imagined she would skydive, but she did. It was a special day. I was absolutely ruined after the three jumps but so glad I did them. Later I found out that Dad thought this was my way of saying goodbye because I was heading back to receive treatment that would be even more intensive than the first. Dr Ganly had used the word 'transplant', and this time we would need to find an unrelated donor because we knew that the bone marrow of my siblings was not a match.

I talked to Clara over the next few days. We had planned for her to come to New Zealand in February 2013, but she decided to come on 1 January. The date seemed far away, but having someone I loved so much, and who loved me, made the second diagnosis more bearable. I would fight for both of our sakes, so we could fulfill our dreams together. Clara gave me hope for a fight that I knew would be so much harder this time. I clung to the belief that within seven months I would be healthy and happy, running and skydiving again, travelling with Clara and fully embracing our life together.

I was wholeheartedly determined to get this fucking cancer job done again, to give it my best fight and learn from every piece of shit it would throw at me; tell the pain over and over that it would not get the better of me, because feeling it meant I was alive. I would prepare myself mentally and embrace it. I would cry and now had someone to cry with. Clara's love held me tight and so strongly. Fortified and confident, I returned to the Bone Marrow Unit, said hello to the nurses again, and my family moved back into Ranui House: all too familiar, but reassuring as I settled in to start my first round of chemotherapy.

A familiar setting

I felt like a seasoned professional, returning to the ward. My nurses were there – Nic, Mikayla, Lizzy, Sarah, Rebecca, Kim and Jayne – all giving me stick, saying, 'Back again, couldn't get enough of us, huh?' And I saw the sadness in their faces. They knew what I was in for, something I didn't yet grasp. Having a bone marrow transplant would be different, a far more intensive treatment.

I told the nurses about all the adventures I'd had since we'd last met: my trip to Nepal, the travels in Asia, meeting Clara, becoming a skydiver. I had not fulfilled all of my dreams, but if I was to die at 25, I would pass away content. Life or death, I would do all I could, all the way. If I died, I would do so after trying my very best to live. Looking back over the 12 months since my first diagnosis I was proud of the decisions I'd made and of all I had done: more than in the rest of my lifetime. Best of all, I had someone special in my life and knew that would help my fight.

My room was the same square box with tight corners. A hamster had more freedom. I had no wheel to run on, just my bed, the basin, shower and toilet. A doctor told me he had a patient who had been to prison, who thought it was worse being in the unit than in a cell with other prisoners.

My nurses came in and out, poking needles, putting up bags of antibiotics, bloods and platelets, and serving my little cup of pills to me like meals: breakfast, lunch and dinner.

As I lay back in my bed at night I heard the all-too-familiar sound of the ticking clock and the clicking of the monitor that my old friend Poley held for me. The sound was more than irritating. Each click told me I was sick, told me I was dying. There was no escaping the torturous tick of the clock or click of the monitor. All I had was my mind, and all I knew was that I had a job to do: get through the shit, get it done, get better and get out.

First round

I received a trial chemical (a new drug in a world-wide study) in combination with two other chemo drugs, to kill off the cancer cells in preparation for the transplant. It was rough. Unlike last time when the sickness came a day or two afterwards, I threw up as soon as they administered it. I knew from the get-go how physically hard this would be. I lay on the bed, crippled and weak, hunched in a fetal position as the all-too-familiar pain returned. And yet this was my fight mode: my body was going to deteriorate, but thoughts of Clara, of holding her, sustained me.

The treatment continued for a month. I became severely neutropenic and spent Christmas and New Year in the isolation room of the Unit. While my mates were celebrating with laughter and fun, I was throwing up in the toilet, constantly fatigued and sore, my muscles and bones aching as if someone had beaten me with a bat. Happy New Year! I saw some of the fireworks in Hagley Park but they did little to cheer me. I was jealous of my friends, angry to be back in hospital, despite realising how blessed I was to have someone so special in my life.

It was hard to maintain focus on the good. The mind returned to its rollercoaster state and that old battle raged within: I was happy then sad, jealous then grateful, back and forth and back and forth. There was so much more going on than the cancer and I tried to learn all I could from this new experience.

Clara is here

The month passed and then on the first of January 2013, Clara walked in my door.

I was ecstatic, and so relieved to hold her, to smell her, like nature itself in its purest form. Her scent was enough to take away the vile taste in my mouth. I felt nothing but a deep love for her. My heart grew. Clara was beautiful. Right away she made a joke about my lack of hair. We laughed, hugged and cried.

Clara was everything to me. Here she was, wearing my favourite dress of hers, barefoot and smiling a smile like a rainbow, glistening white teeth. She gave me hope and energy such as I hadn't felt in nearly a month. My Clara was here. She and my family came to visit every day.

At night, however, I was alone with my thoughts, the monitor on the pump clicking over. My mind was a stuck record playing the same tune over and over. This was my real battle, the constant thoughts: Yes, I'm alive, I have so many good people, then, boom: I want to die, I'm a burden to everyone. The more time I spent alone at night, the deeper I thought about my life and how other people were living theirs. I was tormented by memories.

When I finally slept, I dreamed about running.

I'd always loved running at night, no matter what the weather – rain, cold, no problem. When my mind told me not to go out on those cold, wintry evenings, I resisted it, telling myself I'd enjoy it. I loved the freedom, the joy of running in the gathering dark, watching the sun lower to the horizon, feeling the cold air and my warming body, fingers tingling. I was addicted to those sensations. When I ran, I was at home, surrounded by nature. It was just me, Josh, with no room for worry or self-judgement, my body doing what it did best, in fluid motion. And I'd come home warm, invigorated and content.

Yes, I was a runner. That's the title I identified with. When I ran, the essence of freedom pumped through my veins, filling me with joy. A meditative calm pulsed through my body.

Now my life had changed and that title was gone. No longer a runner, I still craved those moments of intense joy. I had to redefine who I was and find a new title for myself, like 'skydiver' or 'mountain climber'. I was lost and confused over who I was as a person.

And yet my title was there all the time, one I hadn't yet identified with. I would come to learn that the title was 'Josh' and my mission was to find that internal joy and let it flood through my body the way running did – simply by being me and loving myself for who I was, not for what I associated myself with. Only this way would I find peace, acceptance and the small fragments of freedom that I craved so badly.

However, I wasn't there yet, and I'd awaken from these dreams exhausted and crying. The torture continued as I lay in my hospital bed, fully awake. In a pool of sweat. I recalled jumping out of the plane with my friends, the sky my playground with incredible views of the Southern Alps, the pure freedom of the air, and constant happiness. Now here I was locked in my prison, begging in my mind to be where I loved and thrived, not in this shit-box hell-hole spewing up.

Comfort came in my mum's arms with the lunches and dinners she brought in. Hospital meal trays to the Unit often came with mashed potatoes. When the lid came off I would throw up at the mere sight of these piles of white mush. The tea lady, Dot, brought my meals. I always accepted a warm cup of coffee from her, but I could not eat her mashed potatoes. Mum's food was a five-star, three-course meal delivered to my bedside! I was so full of thanks to my wonderful mum and I thanked God for every bite.

After my experience on the balcony at Ranui House, when I wanted to jump, I took care not to fall into an extreme depressive cycle. Clara, Mum, my family, and the techniques I had learned from my counsellor David all helped. I learned to embrace the sadness, frustration and anger as valid emotions, grateful to experience them because they meant I was still alive and breathing. The trick was to use those feelings in a positive way. I focused on all that I loved in life, my passions and desires, achievements and dreams. I stopped asking Why? and concentrated on How? How will I get through this and what can I do for myself that is useful?

Using David's techniques, I told myself it was okay to be negative and that suppressing those feelings would do more harm than good. I wrote in my diary, expressing thoughts with pen and paper. Then I could focus my mind and think of ways to be productive, always moving forward, not backwards, doing what I could and not dwelling on what I could not. If I was lying in bed, I did leg raises. If I wanted to cry, I did. If I felt anger, I let it out and gave myself a pat on the back for all I was accomplishing, rather than feeling guilty and ashamed of all I hadn't done. I thought about what I wanted my future to be like. My mind was changing, determination was growing, I had a higher pain threshold. I fought constantly not to succumb to negative thoughts, to visualise myself as healthy, free, strong and happy.

Chemotherapy was like having your car in first gear, stuck at 10,000 revs, going down little slopes and then struggling up steep hills, the battery never charging. I could not change the situation but could choose my attitude. That was the only thing I had control over.

Clara strolled over to my room from Ranui House every day. She was always a beautiful sight. Some days I couldn't talk and she just sat with me, read her book, or held my hand. It was so simple, having someone next to me, caring for and loving me. Clara made me feel secure.

Mum had been down this road before so she prepared extra food for me and did the little errands for items I needed. Clara didn't have much to do other than visit and I preferred it that way. I didn't want to burden her when she already had pain and sadness. When she offered to help, I'd say, 'No, it's all right,' and that made her feel useless and sad. She eventually told me that this was hard for her. Simply being there to hold my hand was not enough because she loved me so much. Once that was out in the open, I accepted her offers of food and drinks, and thanked her for going back and forth to the supermarket. It helped her feel included in my journey.

My brother and sister visited on the weekends. They teased me and we laughed together. On the days I was allowed out of my room, we shared family meals at Ranui House. I felt blessed to have my family together, helping me through the painful times. Though on this occasion after the first cycle of treatment, one month of being in isolation and a rough chemo regime, I knew this upcoming transplant cycle could definitely kill me, so as a last hurrah, I entered a 5 km run around Hagley Park. Two good mates, Tyler Coll and Andrew Nidd ran with me for support. The race was the hardest I had ever run and I was completely depleted at the finish line, even throwing up. I said goodbye to running with a 26 minute flat chemo-induced run. This was good pain. I smiled as I lay on the ground in the park, content that if I did die I knew I had never given up.

Where has Josh gone?

After three months of treatment, I was nearing my bone marrow transplant date, although they had still not found a donor. There would be a two-month break between the last chemo round and the start of more chemo and radiation before the transplant. Deep down I was anxious about the transplant. The doctors explained that graft vs host disease (GVHD) was a likely side effect. The transplant would give me a new immune system. However, my new immune system could reject my body and GVHD would develop. The disease attacks any tissue in the body – skin, lungs, kidneys, liver, stomach – and can be mild or severe, with the extent of the disease not known until it happens. Dr Ganly said that 70 percent of patients got GVHD and 30 percent died from it. There was a big risk involved, but I had no other option. Without the transplant, I'd certainly die. The GVHD did provide a positive anti-cancer effect: if any cancer cells still remained, my new immune system would attack and kill them. The hope was to get a little GVHD, but not so much that it would kill me.

Ali the transplant coordinator asked if I'd like to speak to someone who had had acute myeloid leukaemia and had also received the allogenic stem cell transplant. The next day a young man walked in my door. Sam Wyatt was in his early 30s and looked so healthy it was hard to believe he'd been so ill. He sat down, smiled, and said, 'It's a fucked-up situation you're in, eh, bro?'

I laughed and nodded. 'Yeah, man,' I said.

I had plenty of questions for Sam. It was reassuring to talk with someone I could relate to so directly, and we both had a good sense of humour. Sam had experienced GVHD for a few months and then it went away. He was no longer on any medication, spent plenty of time in the surf, had travelled through Europe and enjoyed going out for a beer. I would almost certainly have some degree of GVHD. No one could predict how much, but Sam inspired me with his story and I thought, Yep, I'm going to do this, easy-peasy, get it done then go and travel. A little bit of GVHD? No worries!

Sam gave me the confidence to go forward. He was living a normal life post-transplant, the 'new normal' the doctors were always telling me about. His visit lifted my spirits and I was looking forward to the two-month break, going home to Greymouth, breathing the fresh air and taking a drive out the Coast Road. I wanted to show Clara my hometown and all of my favourite places.

'Dad, please kill me!'

A few mornings later, I woke to a searing pain that ripped through my head like lightning exploding. I pushed the buzzer three times. Everything happened fast. Bloods were taken and morphine was given. The pain reduced slightly and I rested for a few hours, then more pain arrived, so intense I began to scream. I'd never felt anything like it. Someone was drilling into my scalp and my brain was burning from the inside out.

I developed a fever. The pain was so bad I wanted to die. Dad came to visit during those excruciating hours. I was curled in a foetal position and screamed at him, 'Dad, please kill me, please!'

I was semi-conscious, pumped full of antibiotics for overwhelming infection and morphine for overwhelming pain. My nurse Rebekah was back and forth, in and out of my room. I have no recollection of what followed, as I was wheeled away to intensive care and placed in an induced coma. I was on life support and a machine was breathing for me. I was in a coma for ten days, long unbearable days for my family and Clara. Only one other person was allowed to visit, my mate Hamish.

The doctors weren't sure I'd wake up. The last round of chemo had destroyed my immune system. It seemed I was dying. Mum and Dad visited every day, holding my hand and talking to me although I couldn't hear them.

I did come back though, slowly but surely, as the doctors managed my situation with care, skill, and numerous bags of antibiotics. I woke to see a collection of doctors surrounding me. 'Josh, can you hear me? Nod if you can hear me.' I nodded, dazed and not knowing where I was. A doctor told me to take a deep breath and they pulled the tube from my throat. I couldn't speak so I was given a white board to write on. I wrote, *Where am I and what happened?*

They told me I was in intensive care and had developed neutropenic sepsis. The chemotherapy had devastated my immune system to the extent that I had contracted a lethal infection. I looked down at my skinny body, far thinner than I remembered. What the fuck just happened? I couldn't comprehend what the doctors were telling me.

It took a while before I got the picture. I was weak, muddled, skinny, with bloodshot eyes and no memory of the previous ten days. My sister had written a diary about my days on life support so I would have an idea of what had happened and how she was feeling.

The focus was always on me, and had been for so long, I often wondered how Rachael and Jacob, were coping. As a young kid, my sister was my best friend and we played 'school', where I was the student and she was the teacher. Rachael is strong, determined, and reading the following words put light into my soul. They made me cry and smile, and I felt so proud of how she had managed, seeing me in such a state. The special relationship she and Jake now share was forged through my suffering. They have a unique bond. Here's what she wrote for me:

Having someone you love go through a battle where there's nothing you can do or say to help, a battle that's completely out of your control, where you have to put your trust in complete strangers, is the hardest thing I've ever had to do. To make it even harder, the person going through this battle was my strong, fit brother, who was always strong for me, always protected me.

One Saturday afternoon Jake and I were on our way to the supermarket so I could buy him some beers for a party that night. Mum called from Christchurch to tell us that Josh was being placed on life support. She told us not to rush over, that we should wait until morning. Jake and I sat outside the supermarket and cried, then he went to be with his friends.

All of my family were away: aunties in Nelson, Mum and Dad with Josh in Christchurch. I was alone and felt sick, not knowing what was happening with Josh. I needed someone to talk to, so I called my best friend Leroy. He was in Christchurch with friends at a party, but did his best to comfort me and get me thinking positively.

Sunday morning Jake and I set out for Christchurch. We sat in silence until we reached the old West Coast Road, then we began to talk. We said things like, 'It's going to be okay', 'It will be just like when Mullet was on life support', 'There will be other people in the room with him', 'We may have to take turns at seeing him'.

As it happened, we both went in with Mum to see Josh.

Nothing could have prepared us for the sight of our seemingly lifeless brother attached to tubes and machines, in his own room, with many doctors coming and going all the time. Jake and I stood back, on either side of the bed. Mum went straight to Josh, took his hand and stroked it, speaking to him softly like the mother of a newborn baby. There was love and fear in her eyes and voice as she watched over her beloved baby. Jake and I shared a look and burst into tears. We couldn't speak to Josh or touch him. We were frozen.

After some time, we got the courage to go closer, to hold his hand and say some words to him. I think Josh knew we were there and could hear us because he tried to open his eyes. We got such a fright the first time that happened.

There were three doctors in the room discussing whether to give him platelets. Josh had had a reaction to the last bag he was given and had needed adrenaline. Again Jake and I looked at each other. What would happen this time? I asked if we should leave the room but the doctors said we could stay.

They gave him the platelets and soon afterwards his body started jerking. I turned to head for the door, only to be stopped by a doctor telling me he was coughing and that it was okay.

Jake had his first day of work on the Monday and I was due back at school for our 'teacher only' days. We wanted to stay longer but the doctors reassured us by saying, 'We're just giving Josh some rest time.' We found out later that Josh had asked the doctors before he was put in a coma to tell us this so we'd continue with our plans.

On the journey home, again, we only started talking at the old West Coast Road. Jake spoke first, saying, 'Mikey said Matt moved too when he was on life support.' (Mike is one of Jake's best friends who had just lost his younger brother Matt). We spent the three-hour journey talking on and off, reassuring each other.

That night we were going to Mike's family's house for dinner. I remember feeling sick with guilt because our brother still had a chance at living, but theirs had lost his life. As we pulled into our drive, our neighbour John Olsen came and asked how Josh was doing. He didn't know about the life support so we filled him in. First thing he did was invite us for dinner but we thanked him, saying we already had plans.

We went to the supermarket to buy something for the dinner and when we got back home there was a $200 petrol voucher at *our front door from the Olsen family. I broke down in tears with Jake at their kindness. At the time I thought it was an odd thing to give us but, looking back, I understand: if Jake and I needed to get back to Christchurch in a hurry, then filling the car up with petrol was taken care of.*

There were so many other acts of kindness. People baked for us, made us meals, and gave us supermarket vouchers. Our Greymouth community showed our family such generosity. It was overwhelming. Now, whenever I feel I can do something to help or support someone in my community, I always try to. I want to pay back the kindness people showed to us by doing the same for others. People will often say to me, 'Rach, you are too kind,' but they don't realise that it was the kindness of others that supported our family through a tough time.

Josh often wonders why Jake and I don't talk much and always jokes that he and I aren't close, but we are. Jake and I have often communicated without words during this time. We have shared many hugs, tears and meaningful glances when we instantly know what the other is thinking. We have a bond that Josh will never understand, a relationship that developed as we sat on the sideline together, watching this battle that Josh has been going through.

I've been hardened by the experience with Josh. When someone says their 85-year-old father-in-law has been diagnosed with cancer, my first thought is, 'Well, he's a lucky bugger to live to 85, and to have children and grandchildren.' If someone is choosing not to look for work, or to turn down a job because they're unhappy with the pay, I think, 'You're bloody lucky you can work.' It annoys me that my first thoughts are like this, but it's because I know Josh would give anything to be able to have these things, and it frustrates me when people take their life and opportunities for granted.

I often grieve for the brother I've lost, the one who was an amazing athlete and could spend his weekend chopping down trees, the one I could party with. Now and then I'll host and attend my own 'pity party', wishing I could be in the stands of QE2 watching Josh run, or listen to a boring story about how he and Hamish dropped x number of trees together. I miss that brother. I knew him well for 21 years. I loved him so much and was so proud of all his achievements.

I'm getting to know my new brother. It's hard, but I am even prouder and more in love with this new man. His opinions, likes and dislikes have changed. His moods can blow hot and cold like the wind. He's different, but then we all are. Watching and being a part of what he has endured over the past several years has been a blessing and a curse. A curse because of the pain, heartache and frustration of watching someone we love go through such suffering. A blessing because we've met so many new people and witnessed first-hand how a positive mental attitude can enhance the healing process. Josh has willingly risked his life taking trial medications, consenting to be a medical guinea pig. I'm in awe of the goals he sets for himself, and reaches. I've seen our family grow stronger, and my eyes have been opened in appreciation of life's simple things.

I'd do anything to take away my brother's pain and suffering. I often cry alone in frustration over the things he has to deal with day by day. I'm so proud of the battle he's fought, and continues to fight, and I'm proud that our family has had the strength to walk the winding road with him. I admire his courage to get out of bed each day, never giving up. There will always be new challenges for him to face. He conquers one, and another appears.

A friend once gave Josh a Crusaders rugby jersey signed by Richie McCaw. Richie wrote on it: 'Sometimes winning is beating the odds.'

You've won so many times on this journey, Josh. You've beaten so many odds, and there are many you haven't shared with us. We used to laugh about this quote before it became real. Now I hold onto it. I hope you'll continue to beat odds and win.

I know there are times when Josh wants to stop taking his

medication, stop treatment and end the suffering. I'm selfish. I'm always hoping and praying that he won't stop. I don't know how our family would survive without him. How selfish of me to think that way.

'We have found you a donor.'

I was so fragile. The nurses sat me up in bed and helped me try to stand. I was too weak, shaking like crazy, unable even to walk by myself.

The first time I saw Clara again with her bright smile I felt like I'd woken from the dead and seen an angel. I was so emotional I wanted to marry her there and then. Clara was my rock, the girl I was determined to live for. Her presence lifted me. Having her in my life, by my side, holding my hand, made me stronger than ever.

Life was the furthest from perfect it had ever been. I was searching hard for the tiniest grains of joy I could find. Seeing Clara again was one of those perfect moments and another was when Dr Steve Gibbons came into intensive care and said, 'We have found you a donor.'

There had been doubts over whether they could find someone. I managed a low and groggy, 'Awesome!' A tear ran down my cheek. I was barely able to speak and still trying to understand where my mind and body had been for the past ten days. An utter mess, I looked like an alien, gaunt face, dark red eyes and skinny little legs. I didn't recognise myself.

The jubilation of hearing I had a donor slowly kicked in and my tears fell. Tears for the pain I had endured and happiness that life was being given back to me, again.

'But,' Dr Gibbons said, 'you have only two weeks to get yourself together before the transplant.'

Two weeks, only two weeks!? I repeated in my scrambled mind. There was supposed to be a two-month break for recovery after a round of chemotherapy, in preparation for further extreme doses of chemo and radiotherapy before the transplant. But this was the only time my donor was available to donate. She had planned her summer vacation and would not be around later. So, there it was. Now or never.

Fuck. My mind went crazy. I couldn't walk, could barely talk. I looked like an alien skeleton. I was so weak I had to be wheelchaired everywhere. How would my body handle the treatment? This was the weakest I'd been in my entire life.

I couldn't even a whisper a reply. There was no other choice. I had to go through with the transplant despite being so tremendously fragile. How would I get well enough in two weeks?

Here I was in the ICU, not talking or walking, as frail as an old man, my mind spinning. I nodded, gave Steve the thumbs-up and said to myself, 'Sweet as.'

Another job to finish.

Preparing for the transplant

Soon enough I was out of the hospital and into Ranui House. I made it my full-time job to recover and gain weight. I had to do all I could for myself because the treatment before the transplant could take my life.

I ate. It was the first time on the cancer journey that I ate crap food. Burger King did the job. I ate as many BBQ Bacon Double Cheese Burgers as I could in two and a half weeks. My brother Jake made the burger run a few times a day. Clara was dismayed by my nutritional choices and I didn't like it either, but I had to put on weight as quickly as possible because the treatment for a transplant is demanding.

I had to ready myself for an allogenic stem cell transplant. The preparatory treatment included six cycles of Total-body irradiation (TBI) combined with high dosage chemotherapy. Toxicity would be extremely high. My doctors told me that some people die from the preparatory treatment alone. My own immune system would not recover. That was the objective. We needed the stem cells from my donor to grow a new immune system. My blood type would change from A+ to O+ and my whole body would change.

I gained a little weight. I sat outside taking deep, healing breaths of clean, fresh air. I pictured every breath healing me from the inside out, filling every cell in my body and I prayed to God to make me stronger before the treatment began.

Although I went to church with the family when I was younger, I never enjoyed it. I didn't fully believe in God but was mildly curious. As I suffered in hospital I had a sense that was new to me, of something bigger than my own life, something stronger than human, as if God was touching me or had my back. I had the sense that God wasn't about rules, but about freedom and love, and that was the essence of it. That's what I held onto. Freedom and love.

The transplant would be hard and I prayed I'd pull through. With an unrelated donor transplant there is a high risk of developing graft rejection, the dreaded GVHD.

My new immune system (the stem cells) was coming from an 18-year-old girl in Germany. That's all I was allowed to know. It was ironic that I had a donor form Germany. Now I had two German angels looking after me. I wrote her a thank-you letter, much of which was edited out by the medical authorities. The postcard I sent featured New Zealand's majestic West Coast so she would have an idea of where I was from. Ali, the transplant coordinator, took this with her when she went to Germany to collect the stem cells.

It was not a perfect match. One of the doctors described it: '… as though we built the same house but the garage was five millimetres off to the left.' That slight difference could mean life or death, and how much GVHD I might acquire was, of course, the unknown. The likelihood of it taking my life was high. The treatment alone could knock me around so hard that I'd be back on life support, fighting for my life again.

Would I ever be the same again?

Life or death: this was my true test. Everything from my past had been building to this moment.

The treatment was extreme, designed to destroy my own immune system to prevent my body rejecting the donor stem cells, and to eliminate any remaining leukaemic cells. The radiation procedure sounded bizarre. I would lie in a box full of rice and be zapped with TBI. After a normal cycle of chemo, blood counts drop and neutrophil levels reduce to zero. Without any infection fighters, the body becomes neutropenic, but after a week or so, the immune system starts to recover.

This time my own immune system would not recover. The stem cells would be grafted in, find their new home in my bone marrow, start producing new red and white blood cells and grow a new immune system. I found the whole thing surreal, trying to comprehend that my new immune system would come from the girl in Germany, and the blood I would bleed in the future would be hers. We'd share the same blood, my new twin and me.

I talked a lot to Clara, who was always supportive. The small things we did made each day special, like walking slowly, sitting in the sun, sipping our coffees or teas, hugging, crying and laughing. I put a lot on her, sometimes maybe too much.

Who was I now? Would I ever be the same again? Would Clara love me if I stayed like this?

To hell and back

The treatment began and it was hellish.

The week of high-dose chemo combined with full-body radiation was killing me from the inside. The feeling of dying, but not actually dying, was mental torture. I was in a semi-coma, dazed, lost. I barely spoke, just uttered a groan now and then.

Clara visited often. She filled my room with love and light. Most days, all I could do was gaze at her smile and fall asleep with the feel of her hand in mine. She gave me purpose and a reason to fight.

The view of Hagley Park sustained me too. By turning my head I could see out the window, watch the wind in the leaves, the sky and clouds. I was in a dream state, in and out of myself, losing touch. I could speak only in fragments: 'Please, drink', or 'Thank you', then put my head back on the pillow in utter exhaustion as if I'd run 25 km in the hills at a 100-metre pace. It felt as if my body was crumbling, my soul being sucked out. My mind was fuzzy, playing the same, painful record over and over.

I longed to be outside like everyone else – walking, smiling, laughing and pain-free. I couldn't talk about the things my friends were doing because my life had become so different to theirs. My room had become my world. When I was in there, I wanted out, and when I was out, I missed my 'safe' house. The isolation room was my house. If I was sick, help came right away. Away from there, I became scared, even though I was outdoors and in my favourite places. I would feel like a lost and scared little boy wandering aimlessly in the park, utterly exhausted.

This time, though, there was no getting out. Not too many friends visited because of the strict isolation. Only my family and Clara.

The arrival of the cells

The stem cells arrived within the 92 hours after my last cycle of chemo and radiation. The cells were frozen in the special container Ali kept beside her on the flight. Seven of them, a good number, were infused through my Hickman line, quick and painless. Stem cells know where to go. They work their way into the bone marrow and start producing immune cells.

My family, Clara and I had been waiting weeks for this moment but it was short lived. One hour later the bag of stem cells was empty and the excitement in the room had gone. Now I had to lie and wait nervously to see if the cells would accept my body.

The nurses teased me. Mikayla knew I had a female donor and

asked, 'When will you start growing breasts, Josh?' She always knew how to put a smile on my face.

After a few days I became very ill, spewing and shitting up to 30 times a day. It was horrendous. My nurse Nic said I had acute GVHD in my gastrointestinal tract. My shit was vile. Green, stringing liquid. The smell was terrible and my stomach was torn apart again.

My nurses had always been my heroes and I admired them even more now that I had become a baby, struggling to walk, shitting my bed, vomiting constantly, the worst episode since my diagnosis. I wore diapers. The nurses wiped my bum like a little kid. I was too weak to object or do it myself.

I was on a pump with multiple bags of antibiotics, food, fluids, steroids and immune-suppressant drugs. They gave me everything my body needed. I lay on my bed in complete exhaustion, holding onto my visualisations, trying to smile, but even that was sometimes too hard. The nurses took care of my needs, bringing cups of water with straws so I could sip, feel the coolness in my mouth, then spit out into another cup. They brought mouth-wash, and brushed my teeth for me.

Because of the delicate state of my stomach, I wasn't allowed to eat or swallow. The highlight of each day was lemonade. Mum, Clara or one of my nurses would bring two cups and put the straw between my lips. I'd take a sip and let the bubbles snap and crackle inside my mouth. The *pop pop pop* in my mouth was a delight, a simple joy. I smiled quietly for that brief moment, then drifted back into a deep sleep with the satisfaction of bubbles in my mouth.

Life can give such small, intense pleasures when you have nothing else. Bubbles popping in my mouth.

Three months of isolation

I couldn't eat for three months. I was fed through an IV. I visualised and prayed every day, for life, and to leave my isolation room.

Once again, I felt as if I was dying, as if my body was shutting down. I was on high doses of morphine for the continual pain. Every little movement made my whole body ache, as if I'd fallen down a cliff. The morphine barely eased the discomfort, but it helped put me to sleep and take me to that semi-comatose dream state.

Eyes closed, I pictured myself free, running, skydiving, rigging up a power line with the boys, or simply holding Clara's hand and walking through a paddock, barefoot in the lush, long grass, sun warm on our faces.

I thought of people worse off than me. I'd seen young children in Nepal sitting on the streets, homeless, no mother, trying to feed themselves. I'd read several books about World War II and thought about the people who suffered in the concentration camps, living through starvation, abuse and extreme cold winters. I had a bed, could hold my mum's hand, feel Clara's fingers in mine, and I had fizzy bubbles popping in my mouth. Yes, I was suffering, but I was being cared for and I was in the right place.

The days passed slowly. I stayed in my half-asleep state, on my sweat-soaked hospital bed, completely exhausted. I don't remember much: just Clara, Mum, Dad, Rach and Jake, the nurses, and the bubbles.

I often wondered if I would live through the night and wake up the next day. I hovered in a limbo-land between life and death. I was conscious enough to know I was dying and had endless thoughts, not about a 'bucket list' or wishing I had a million dollars in the bank, but rather about the person I was, the people I loved, how I acted and reacted in certain situations.

Why was I such a dick to that person? Why didn't I love someone for who they were? Why didn't I give them my all?

I sat in judgement, analysing my life, weighing up the good and the bad, like God. I sought forgiveness, made a vow to survive and be the best version of myself I could be. If I lived, I had to love with respect and empathy. I had to learn from every person who stepped into my life. If I was going to die, I wanted to go knowing I had done all I could to show love for the people I cared about. I wanted to love and forgive myself too.

I often looked out the window and stared at beautiful nature, telling myself I'd feel the wind soon. I watched the trees and the leaves blowing, the people walking by, and I imagined myself as a tree standing tall and strong, feeling the air on my naked skin. I drifted back into deep sleep, holding visions inside my head that I would live.

Tasja

Around that time, a young Greymouth girl Tasja Murphy was diagnosed with a rare brain tumour, metastatic choroid plexus papilloma, scary stuff for her mum and dad. Tasja was two years old and endured two brain surgeries and six months of chemo, also in Christchurch hospital. Her parents Phil and Tash would push her past my window and wave to me. My heart sank every time because that beautiful little girl was going through all this shit. Her treatment was different to mine and no less difficult. She was a resilient wee girl who had the most brutal start to her life. I imagine young children don't really understand what is going on. Of course, the treatment is painful and uncomfortable, but perhaps they think it is normal, as they have little to compare it to.

I wondered if I should think the same and tell myself this was normal. Soon I'd be allowed to go and play, be a kid, cry, laugh, and engage with small things, make a complete game out of a soft toy and use my imagination to take me away from here.

This two-year old girl taught me a different way of approaching my situation. She reminded me of being young, when I built other worlds in my imagination. During those endless days in my isolation room, I constructed castles in my head, whole worlds where I could go and live a fairytale life.

We're all students in life. We never learn enough, though we can't learn everything.

I wrote a note to Tasja's parents, saying how much I felt for them and their wee daughter, and that their love for her would be the strongest and most powerful gift they could give. My ability to have kids was gone. I couldn't begin to understand how a parent must feel, but I knew what cancer felt like, and so a connection grew.

Tasja is now five and full of life. Her happiness and cheeky manner is infectious. I visit her often and all her school friends call me her 'boyfriend'. Her fight to be in this world has made her one special kid.

Freedom

After three months my isolation ended and I walked out a free man. No more chemo, ever. I was free from the isolation room, the pumps and the monitors, the death-tick of the clock and that sterile alcohol environment. Now I could start to heal this body of mine.

GVHD didn't let me go so easily. My skin was bright red, my face puffed up like a balloon from the high-dose steroids. I walked like an old man, bent over, tired and weak. The GVHD had attacked my mouth and I had raw, painful ulcers. Eating solid foods hurt too much.

I stayed at Ranui House for months, until the GVHD was manageable. 100 days was the magic number. We would know by then if the GVHD was turning from acute to chronic.

Every organ in my body was vulnerable to attack from my new immune system. I was released on high-dose steroids and antihistamines, cyclosporine (a drug to suppress the immune system, preventing it from functioning fully and thereby reducing the risk of attack), and heaps of antibiotics and antiviral medications since my infant immune system was susceptible to every pathogen, bacteria and virus.

As an outpatient I received daily 'top-ups' of blood, magnesium, and potassium. Even though I was eating well, my body struggled to absorb minerals and vitamins from the food and I easily became depleted of nutrients. My body was working overtime, as if it had run fifty 100-km races.

'What the fuck did you just do to me?'

I made two good friends at Ranui House: Brian Bell and Derrick Compton. Brian was receiving treatment for mantle cell lymphoma. His own stem cells were collected, and infused back into his body after chemo, in what is called a 'self-rescue' or autologous stem cell transplant. We hung out a lot. Brian was older, a really good man, a down-to-earth soul, a farmer who loved sport and having a good laugh and a bit of mischief. We talked on a deeper level and shared our belief in God, sport, hard work and the beauty of the New Zealand bush and mountains where we both felt free.

Brian and I shared our thoughts about our finances. When you are sick the bills do not stop, but your income does – food, mortgages, insurances, rates still have to be paid and for some people they have a business to run. We were both so grateful to be staying at Ranui House for free. We agreed that not only were we affected but so were our families who were supporting us. Money is a concern for most families staying at Ranui House – money is not everything but when you are sick you definitely appreciate having a job and an income.

Brian and I often took walks together through Hagley Park, discussing our battles with the mind, those voices in the head that get out of control, and how you lose yourself at night when the head touches the pillow, into the nightmares, the vivid dreams. Brian knew about the constant voices, back and forth in your head, about wanting to die then wanting to live, the uncertainty of life, the financial battle. We talked about all of these things and made jokes about how ugly we looked. Brian was jealous of me as he thought I was the nurses' favourite patient. Even older men can act like sulky kids.

One afternoon Brian and I were sitting downstairs watching the cricket at Ranui House. It was a hot summer day and a cold drink sounded good. We decided to take a walk to the gas station down the road. Being determined and stubborn, we set out on our walk, but it was way too far. We were absolutely ruined by the time we got there. We were sweating like we'd had a shower while our bald heads glowed in the sun and drooped towards the ground. What a sight we must have been, sitting there with our bottles of water, looking like two junkies who'd been sniffing fumes. We barely made it back.

I slept for a week afterwards, in serious pain from headaches, with my body screaming, 'What the fuck did you just do to me?' My mind remembered what I was able to do in the past, but the body was different now. Adjusting was another battle in itself.

Derrick was from Golden Bay and had been diagnosed with acute myeloid leukaemia too. He also had allogenic stem cell treatment from a foreign donor, though not the same chemo and radiation. In his early 60s, Derrick talked about his place up in Golden Bay where he could almost launch his boat from his house, he lived so close to the ocean. We made a deal that Clara and I would come and visit.

We often talked about our time in hospital. Although we had the same type of cancer with different markers, our treatment protocols varied. No two patients are the same, but we both understood the pain, the sheer agony of it all.

I needed to keep my mind occupied so resumed study for the photography diploma I had started at skydiving school. I spent the days photographing ducks, sitting outside the boat shed on the Avon River, a beautiful setting opposite Ranui House. I sipped coffee and watched people walk by. I took small walks with Clara and had short outings with Dad at night, walking 100 metres down the road and back. I was careful to do only as much as my body could handle.

My body goes crazy and Ranui House is full of saviours

Ranui House was an absolute blessing and safe haven. To have a home so close to the security of the hospital was ideal, especially when things started going on in my chest.

After the transplant, my body went crazy sometimes and the doctors didn't always know why. I began having frequent chest pain, sharp and stabbing. It would drop me to the ground. There were many 3 am hospital visits to the emergency department with Clara to get 100 mg of IV morphine for pain relief. Clara was a strong girl.

When the pain came, she put me on her shoulder and off we'd go.

On one occasion, Clara had gone out for groceries. That time, I rang downstairs for help. The receptionist shot up in a flash, put me in the wheelchair stationed outside my room and sprinted across to the hospital. Clara and I joked about the constant running back and forth. We laughed over how crazy it was and wondered what on earth would happen next. I had all kinds of tests to find out what was causing the chest pain. Nothing showed up and the attacks continued, week after week. I felt like a burden and it was exhausting for both of us. This was not the life Clara expected or deserved and I hated what I was doing to her. The pain did have a purpose, however. It strengthened our relationship, and her love and care for me were clear. After five months the persistent pain stopped, just like that.

One morning Clara made me a bowl of muesli for breakfast. She'd added fruit, including kiwifruit. She was working down the road at a car wash company, so she went off to her job and left me on my own.

As I ate, my body started to react strangely. I started feeling warm, my skin became red, my breath began to fade and my chest hurt. Fuck. I had to get help. I staggered out the door and collapsed in the corridor. Fortunately Helen, one of the Ranui House cleaners, was coming out of the elevator. She picked me up, put me into a wheelchair and ran me over to the hospital A and E. I was coughing, struggling for air, dizzy and confused. The nurses took me straight in because they knew I was a having an anaphylactic reaction – but to what? Oxygen mask, medication, I could breathe again. I was back.

Helen was a true champion. She helped save my life.

I took an allergy test. They placed a small drop of kiwifruit extract on my skin and as soon as it hit, the area swelled up, so we had found the culprit.

Simple pleasures

The simplest things brought me such pleasure. I had my camera, Clara, and my constant longing to be outside. Clara and I often took little trips to the beach where we'd sit and talk. My mates visited. It was always hard to talk about my health, but I enjoyed seeing their faces.

Hamish was living in Christchurch with his partner Amy. She became good friends with Clara and the two went rock climbing together. I was glad Clara had a mate to hang out with.

Clara introduced me to yoga. We sometimes went to a yin yoga class, where the poses were less stressful and held for five minutes. I loved it, but struggled a lot. My body was so tight and stiff, it was nice to feel 'good pain' in a deep stretch, to relax my mind and concentrate on my breath. I loved the end of the practice where we lay on our backs and did a meditation. This was the calmest I had been in months. Yin yoga was perfect for me: it was difficult but I could hold the poses for as long as I felt comfortable and rest as much as I liked, so when Clara went rock climbing I stayed at Ranui House, stretched, and focused on my breathing.

I was still very weak and couldn't function too well. There is indeed such a thing as 'chemo brain' and my memory was poor. Clara would often find yoghurt or milk in the oven that I'd put there thinking it was the fridge. Notes were everywhere, reminders to 'Have a shower' and 'Brush your teeth' because I forgot the simplest things.

Clara and I have an adventure

As beautiful as Christchurch was, I longed for Greymouth. I was still under constant monitoring by the doctors and wasn't allowed to leave the city. I knew that had to be. It was nice to have Hagley Park across the road from Ranui House, but I needed my home. I wanted to sit with Clara on the beach, show her my place and soak up that West Coast goodness. She and I planned a secret escape for the weekend. The doctors would be none the wiser. It was mid-winter. Dad was staying at Ranui House with us and I was tired of him being around. I needed a break. Clara and I would sneak off, take the train to Greymouth and see the snow at Arthur's Pass.

On a cold, brisk morning Clara and I woke up and waited for Dad to leave for work. The coalmine he worked at had recently closed down and he'd taken a part-time contract in Christchurch as an electrician, staying with Clara and me at Ranui House.

As soon as he left, we grabbed the bags we'd packed the night before and made our way to the train station. I was breaking the rules. A schoolkid excitement and rush of adrenaline went through my blood, as it had at skydiving school. We boarded the train and we were off.

I felt free again, attached to nothing but Clara, off on an adventure. I had called my brother and asked him to leave a car at the Greymouth train station so we could surprise Mum at work. I couldn't wait to see the look on her face.

I went to the viewing platform as we approached Arthurs Pass. It was a clear, cold winter's day. I felt the icy air touch my face, my friend the wind all around me. I closed my eyes and embraced every bit of it, picturing the wind wrapping around my body and healing me. I was home. The snow on the slopes was magnificent, so clear and pure. Memories of Nepal flooded back and I remembered the feel of the wind at skydiving school, jumping from a plane at 12,000 feet.

I was overwhelmed and cried with joy that I was still alive and breathing. Even though I'd seen all the beautiful rugged scenery many times before, this was like seeing it for the first time. As the train ploughed through the snow, I let out a wolf cry of delight, feeling every sensation through my body. No one could take this moment from me.

We arrived in Greymouth, found the car and drove to Mum's work. We walked in with big grins on our faces, knowing we were doing something wrong, but it felt so good.

Mum looked up. At first she looked surprised, then angry and a bit sad, and finally she started to cry. 'What are you doing here?' she kept asking. We were laughing like kids, hugging her and I said, 'It's okay, Mum. I had to see you and my beautiful Greymouth.'

I assured her I had all my medication and morphine just in case and she cried more happy tears. We had a nice dinner with Mum, Rachael and Jacob.

Ruth's dad owned a trucking company and we got a ride back to Christchurch the next day in one of his trucks. My friend Tyler was driving. The journey was a slow one and I'll never forget driving up Porter's Pass and seeing the sun rise. The early morning sunshine lit up the pass like a snowy heaven, glistening like millions of diamonds. The hills where alive and talking to me.

I needed that adventure. I returned to Ranui House fulfilled and happy, holding onto the memories of snow, wind, sunrise and shining hills, the look of surprise on Mum's face, the delight of seeing my brother and sister again.

My skydiving friends Matt, Iohann and Wayne visited often at Ranui House. They kept me up to date on the goings-on at school, told me about their jumps and I longed to play in the sky with them, but I was too weak.

The glimpse into my life as it had been made me want to skydive again, to run and to travel, but I knew it served no purpose to dwell on all the things I was missing out on, so I closed my eyes and embraced those fun moments and memories of jumping out of planes, running with the wind and travelling to exotic places. There were always tears of envy because I longed to be far from where I was. I wiped them away, picked myself up and thought, Soon Josh, soon. You'll be back.

At the time of my first diagnosis, I had suffered, tormenting myself over all I had lost. The disappointment of not winning gold at the NZ Champs had been so raw and all but consumed me. I changed my thinking and told myself how blessed I was to have accomplished so much. I was a fast runner and that was great. I was a skydiver and that was awesome. I had been to Nepal and adventured around Asia. I drew strength from my past. I was living life and it was full, even if I never ran or jumped again. I held onto my dreams and was more accepting of what was possible and what might not be, and if I was never able to do those things again, at least I had experienced them.

It was no longer about being the best, rather simply being a part of it, making friends, accepting the support I had been so fortunate to receive, sharing stories with my friends and family. This was the real achievement and my next one would simply be to stay alive and live.

I continued on with a clearer head and a deep love for Clara. I would get myself back to where I wanted to be. Of that I was sure.

Home at last but steroids wreak havoc

After nearly a year at Ranui House I returned home to Greymouth. It was November 2013, the roller coaster ride of being trucked back and forth to the hospital was over, my body was slowly accepting the graft and the GVHD was under control with medication. There was always the potential for the GVHD to become chronic and I would have monthly check-ups for the foreseeable future.

Our family home was full, with no room for Clara and I, so my Auntie Irene let us stay in her holiday house on Tahuna Beach in Nelson. Summer was on the way and it was a perfect place to recover. Nelson served me well and we stayed there for three months. My body grew stronger and I was able to decrease my medications.

Our time was simple yet fulfilling. We ate good food, went for walks along the beach, practiced yoga together, talked and laughed about the circus act of shipping me back and forth from Ranui House, all of the antics I'd pulled during my transplant, and waking up from life support. It was a nice, easy time.

It was refreshing to breathe the clean air, with no hospital monitors clicking away or nurses waking me up at 3 am for observations, no morphine, just Clara's hand in mine and the ocean breeze on our faces. The crazy, mad times were fading. Mum, Dad, Rachael and Jake visited on the weekends.

That year of my transplant had been madness and I felt such gratitude for how far I'd come since then and all of the people who'd helped me. I'd raise my hand up, squeeze a tight fist and watch the arteries pulse beneath my skin. The blood filling my veins came from the stem cells of a young girl. I was half woman! I had also received over 50 bags of blood and platelet transfusions during the course of my treatment and I was grateful for the generosity of the people who had donated their blood and given me life. I wished I had been a donor during my fit and healthy years and known what a gift that could be to someone. I thanked God for the breath of life and the kindness of strangers.

The downside was the high dose of steroids I had to take. I hated it. The steroids threw my moods all over the place. I was up and down like a yo-yo: angry, sad, extreme and out of control. I yelled and screamed at my family over nothing, then burst into tears. The meds made me feel hungry all the time and I ate like crazy. That was good because I needed the nutrition.

Steroids can have vicious side effects, destroying eyes and muscles, affecting bone density, and more. Physically, I still felt weak, fragile, and was often depressed. Some days I thought the bad effects outweighed the good. The two main medications were the steroids and the cyclosporine. Dr Ganly and I were working towards a goal of 'zero meds', carefully decreasing the dosage of the steroids while trying to find a level that would still be effective for the GVHD, and which I could handle better mentally.

The sight in my left eye was diminishing and a check-up confirmed that a cataract had developed as a side effect of the high-dose steroids. I knew the medication served an important purpose, but it was taking life from me. My bones and muscles ached, my mind was all over the place, my emotions were uncontrollable at times, and my strength was fading, so I was determined to get off the nightmarish pink prednisone pills.

I'd heard horror stories of people on high doses of prednisone. Their bones had been weakened to such a degree that some had broken their backs and been confined to wheelchairs. That was not going to happen to me. I spent time researching the effects of steroids on the human body so I could make well-informed choices.

During our stay at Tahuna Beach, I had plenty of time and freedom to be alone and think. I often thought of the other patients I'd met. Some had better prognoses than I did and yet they'd passed away. Some had worse. I had grown close to these people. We had shared our pain and I struggled when they died. I remember one young boy whose name I can't recall.

I met him at Ranui House after my second diagnosis. He attended Christ's College and was exceptionally bright. Around 1 o'clock one morning, I went to the communal room to make a cup of tea and he was sitting on the couch watching TV. I sat down with him and we started talking. The weather is the least popular topic of conversation in a cancer house so we talked about our disease. He told me he had only weeks to live because they couldn't find a donor. I was astonished. How could this be? I wanted to give him my stem cells.

He explained that his cancer had progressed far beyond any chance of rescue.

I was lost for words and there was no way I could return to my room so I walked around the block, breathing in the fresh air, feeling sad, angry and frustrated that life was being taken from this young boy.

I wish that I'd asked him to walk with me. I wish I'd said more than just, 'I'm sorry,' because 'sorry' doesn't cut it sometimes.

Now, when I'm lost for words, I hug.

I hug them tight and say how much I love them.

My good Ranui House friend Derrik Compton had a transplant like me. He passed away while I was in Nelson. He was in his 60s. His wife Annette called me the day before he died, and said, 'Derrick wants to speak with you. He's not too good.' Derrick's voice was weak and husky. I sensed the life draining from him. He told me he might die soon. I clung to every whispered word he said. We shared a small giggle and then his voice became stronger and firmer. 'Josh, I love you,' he said.

I shared those words back to him, hung up the phone and cried tears of sadness that I had lost a good friend, and tears of joy that Derrick's suffering was ending. I was grateful for the time we had shared together.

Clara's family

Clara and I were enjoying our new-found freedom when we received an email from her sister saying she, husband Lucas and their wee boy Noah were coming over to travel about in a campervan for a few months. The rest of the family would join us for Christmas – Klaus, Sabine, Jan and his partner Moni. All would be hopping into vans and tripping around the South Island.

Clara and I had often talked about taking a road trip so we decided to join the fun.

We purchased a Toyota Town Ace. I wasn't strong enough to fit it out myself so I drew up a design and a local joiner in Nelson did the work. It turned out great: comfortable with lots of room.

Right after the New Year we hit the road. The van was perfect because when we reached our destination, I could rest and relax in the back while the family went on their walks. It was no stress for me and Clara was delighted to have her family around her after such an up-and-down year. We shared our experiences with her family. They were astonished to hear of all we had endured.

It did me so much good to be with her family. They were humble, generous people who cared deeply for each other. I felt privileged to be a part of them. All too soon they returned to Germany and Clara and I were left to ourselves again.

And now . . . a word from my donor

I had to decide what to do with myself. A part-time job? Study? I'd found in the past that when I started thinking about my life, events were set in motion and life would throw up opportunities I had never expected.

My two past running mates, Hayden McLaren and Matt Lambert, were House Supervisors at Nelson Boys High School. The 2014 school year was starting and they knew of an opening for a supervisor in one of the boarding houses, Rutherford House. Hayden and Matt thought it would be the perfect job for me so they asked if I was interested.

I would supervise the boys after school from 3 until 5 pm, and then spend a few nights after dinner helping them with homework. I would receive accommodation, food and time to myself. The job would not be strenuous and Clara could join me.

I got the job. The boys in Rutherford House were fun to be around and found their way into my heart. I knew that school didn't always set you up for life's hardships and changes so I tried to instill some sound values into the boys, developing good, positive relationships with them. I still keep in contact with a handful of boys, watching with interest as they progress in their life journeys.

I picked up a part-time job in the weekends driving the van for Skydive Motueka, bringing tourists from Nelson to the drop zone. I loved being part of a team again and even managed a few jumps when my body was up to it. I was so grateful to have some normality back, and being involved with people who were not hospital-related helped distract my mind from the past year.

One day the receptionist from Skydive Motueka contacted me to say she had received an email from my donor. I couldn't believe it because communication between donor and recipient was not encouraged. There had been occasions when a donor or recipient had taken advantage of the situation with a 'You owe me now' type approach. Consequently, parties involved were given little opportunity to learn much about each other.

I had written to my donor at the time, sending that thank-you card with a picture of the majestic West Coast on the front. I told her I was a skydiver, but the Bone Marrow registry had edited out the rest of my personal details. My donor had done some investigating and found me.

In her email she said her name was Hannah. She was 19 years old and lived in Germany. She knew I was a skydiver and the photo indicated I was probably in the South Island, so she emailed all the southern skydive centres, asking if anyone had recently had cancer and a transplant. Of course no one had, except for me. Hannah and I began emailing back and forth, getting to know one another. I was so curious to know more about her. Did we look at all the same? Act the same? It was truly incredible, unbelievable in fact, that we were in contact. It was so exciting to hear from this kind-hearted girl who had saved my life. We talked about meeting one day.

Coping with 'the new normal'

My body was doing well despite the fatigue and pain. I exercised and ate the food I needed to rebuild my weak body. Nearly a year since my transplant I was still short of my normal weight of 68 kg, just holding onto 61 kg.

The recovery took far longer this time and was more strenuous. There was no way I could have made it to Base Camp. My body was different and I was trying to find my way through the 'new normal' that the doctors and nurses always talked about.

'I'll show them,' I said in my head. 'I'll get back to myself.'

I felt different on the inside too, like someone had torn my skin off and put it on a new body. I was 26, waking up stiff, sore and groggy every day, fighting on a daily basis to get my body to do what my mind wanted. Not always possible.

Some days, which were most days, I felt so old, weak and fragile, as if my friend the wind could pick me up and sweep me away. Those were the tough days, when I thought I wasn't getting better, when I felt lost and frustrated, unable to acknowledge that, overall, I was slowly getting stronger. The mind is a beast that is hard to tame, and all I could do was focus on what I loved dearly.

Clara worked part-time at an orchard that summer. As the season neared its end, we made some plans. We agreed she should start university in Germany. I would travel over at the end of the school year. We had been through so much together and felt that our relationship was strong enough to weather time apart. Clara had been by my side since the start of 2013 and now was her chance to do something for herself.

She left New Zealand in May 2014. Even though we knew we'd

see each other soon, the separation was tough. Clara was the one who had always been there and now she was on the other side of the world, establishing a life in Berlin, studying social work. We spent a lot of time on Skype.

As time went by I grew stronger at Nelson Boys. By November, I was fit and well enough to travel. I walked through the airport doors in Berlin and there she was, standing with a grin on her face. We embraced each other as lovers. It was as though we hadn't been apart.

Berlin in winter

Berlin was ice cold, a tough winter for someone in my condition. I was still on moderate doses of steroids and immune suppressants. I had gained weight, was looking and feeling good, but was unprepared for the cold.

It was wonderful to be with Clara and we were happy. I helped to decorate her little apartment that was not much bigger than my isolation room.

Berlin is an exciting, incredible city with so much history. I had always been interested in World War II and embraced my time in Berlin, visiting as many historical sites as I could.

I felt for the people living in such a big city. The buildings in West Berlin were beautiful from the outside but in the East they were like rat cages. I couldn't understand how people lived like that, no freedom, bunched into apartments like sardines, no park close by to escape into nature.

My donor Hannah and I had been emailing before my trip and when I told her I was visiting Germany, we decided to meet. She was studying at a university one hour by train from Berlin, an easy journey for me to make.

Hannah sent a photo so I would know her when I arrived. Everyone thought she looked more like a sister to me than Rachael and I wondered how similar we actually were, considering we now had the same blood type (mine had changed from A+ to Hannah's O+) and immune system.

It seemed surreal that I was going to meet her. Clara came with me and on the way we talked about how lucky I was because most patients don't get the opportunity. Besides which, some donors aren't interested in meeting them.

We arrived at the train station full of nerves and a tad scared. Hannah was waiting with a huge smile. We all hugged and I cried. I didn't even say hello. All I could say was 'Thank you', again and again.

We went to Hannah's apartment and sat down for a decent chat. Hannah was a delightful, down-to-earth girl, genuine and happy. She had a deep appreciation of life and was not taking hers for granted. She told us that being a donor was really no big deal. The bone marrow registry in Germany visited her school, asking for donors. A handful of students signed up and agreed to a saliva swab for DNA. Hannah was surprised at how quickly they had contacted her to be my donor.

She travelled to a special centre in Dresden to have her stem cells drawn.

'Was it a tough process?' I asked.

'It was easy,' she said. 'They gave me some medication to stimulate my immune system. I felt like I had a cold. It was really no problem.'

Hannah had stayed in Dresden for a week with her aunt and received injections of granulocyte colony stimulating factor (G-CSF). This stimulated her stem cells to enter the blood stream. Once there were enough peripheral blood stem cells (PBSC) in her blood stream, Hannah was attached to a blood separator (apheresis machine), the cells were extracted, collected and sent to me.

I was in awe of the young woman who had done all this for me. I listened to all she had to say, watching her intently, all the while thinking that this girl was my sister, in a way. We shared the same DNA and blood. I was a kind of replica of her. It was a real mind-blower.

I was glad Clara was there because I barely spoke, lost for words, overwhelmed by the generosity of this girl who had saved my life, and by the fact of actually meeting her. We had a nice dinner together and visited a German Christmas market.

I thank Hannah every day from the bottom of my heart. Hannah's family and mine keep in contact, and her younger sister came to visit us in February 2017.

The connection is close and special.

The New Year: 2015

Clara and I stayed with her parents in Schloss Hamborn over Christmas and New Year. The continual cold took a toll on my health. I started coughing, spitting up gobs of green phlegm the size of squash balls. Then blood started coming up too. I thought it was just a chest infection. I was still taking penicillin, antivirals and antibacterial medication so figured it would soon pass.

Two days later we were on our way back to Berlin with Clara's brother Jan and his partner Moni. I got out of the car and collapsed. Jan was worried and wanted to take me straight to hospital. The voice in my head was shouting, Fuck no, please, not the hospital! I wanted to be with Clara and establish myself here with her, to forget about illness. I wanted a peaceful life with the woman I loved. I'd had my transplant and wanted nothing more to do with hospitals.

But I had to go. I'd developed pneumonia and spent a week in Berlin Hospital. Here I was, all over again, Clara coming to visit, bringing me food. It was déjà vu.

Looking back on it, I have to laugh. They didn't have a bed available in a ward so I spent the first two nights in the supply room with all the medication. I couldn't believe they put me in there with full access to all these medicines. They didn't know me. I could've grabbed all the pills I wanted. The nurses kept coming in and out and I never got any sleep. Finally I was taken to a room and put on IV antibiotics.

It was frustrating and sad. Clara and I knew I had to go home, sort myself out in the New Zealand summer, regain my strength and return to her when I was better.

It was heart-wrenching to leave her. There were floods of tears but we both knew that the Berlin winter was too harsh for me. I was too weak and had to get well. We would try again in summer.

Back to New Zealand

I came home, rested and regained some strength.

Kim, one of my nurses, was doing a bike ride around Lake Brunner to raise money for the NZ Leukaemia and Blood Cancer Foundation. One night in hospital when I'd been very sick, Kim and I had promised we'd ride together. I never break my word so we dubbed this ride 'a promise is a promise'. Although I was still weak, I wanted to ride and managed to bike the last few kilometres as part of the team. Dr Peter, some other doctors and nurses, my good friend Ruth, and Rachael and Jacob rode with us. Once again, it was déjà vu, crossing the finish line at Lake Brunner. It felt great to be giving back, supporting a good cause, and afterwards I was exhausted.

I had to ask myself why I pushed so hard and did things when I wasn't ready. I'd always fought for everything I did, sometimes to my detriment. Still, it felt good being part of the team, if only for the last little bit.

Love rules

Recovery went well. I was in the gym and eating the food I needed. I loved Mum's cooking, good whole foods, lamb roast and vegetables. I had tried a vegetarian and vegan diet the year before, experimenting with different foods, but felt better when I was eating fatty meat like lamb and pork. I put on weight but deep down I knew I needed at least two more years to get myself in good shape physically and mentally. Although my GVHD was stable on the medication, I wasn't yet back to where I wanted to be.

Clara called to say she missed me and that I must return to Germany.

Love pulls us in all directions, even when we're not ready. Love rules. That's all there is to it.

When I felt something deep inside, I pursued it, because it had purpose for me. If someone told me, 'Man she's hot, go for it!' or 'You need to be doing this,' I wouldn't do it. I had to feel it for myself, from my heart and in my head, then I'd do it.

I felt so much for Clara, my girl. She was with me when I woke from the coma, held my hand when I was sad, hugged me, wiped my tears, literally carried me to the hospital in the early hours of the morning when I had horrendous chest pain. I loved her for all she'd done for me. Clara, and love, were calling.

I wasn't 100 percent ready for travel, and returning to Germany wasn't the smartest plan. How ready or smart do you have to be? I wasn't fully recovered but knew if I didn't go, I'd regret it for the rest of my life. I had to try. I'd been on my deathbed, thinking about life, the should-haves and wouldn't-haves, every fine detail, judging, evaluating, criticising, wishing I'd been that 'other' kind of person and had made different choices. I didn't want to die knowing that I hadn't tried.

I loved this girl and that was life to me. Love.

Germany again – the same, but different

In April 2015 I endured the agonising 32-hour flight to Berlin. I was exhausted when I arrived, sweat running down my face, eyes bloodshot, body shaking, in desperate need of sleep. Seeing Clara's face was like the sight of a wondrous bloom, always new and beautiful no matter how many times it is seen.

I decided to make the most of my time, embrace the German language, settle in and do my best to recover away from the security of my doctors at home. I went into the city, spoke to as many people as I could, enrolled in a language school and after three months was having short conversations. Learning something new engaged and fascinated me and I picked up enough German to get around alone with confidence.

Things were different with Clara, though. I thought maybe

university life had changed her. Maybe she had experienced how good life can be without the burden of worrying and looking after a sick, weak old man like me. Clara became more withdrawn and not as open as she had been. Maybe life in Berlin with all its excitement and attractions had broadened and changed her thinking. I didn't think too much of it at the time. All I knew was that this wasn't the same girl I fell in love with.

Clara's tiny apartment was congested with two of us there, so I had to give her space because I knew she was confused and unsure about me being there.

I went out a lot, throwing myself wholeheartedly into the culture of the city. It was summer. I rode a bike to the nearest park and set up my slackline, like a tightrope but 'slack', tied between two trees. I walked the line, concentrating on my breathing and giving my body much-needed movement, then I'd sit down in the shade to meditate, think, write and study the German language. The park was my sanctuary and nature was my calling. The cigarette butts littering the ground reminded me I was still in a city but I could sweep them away, find my own green patch of grass and call it mine. I was grateful for my freedom every minute of every day. I was outside where fresh air filled my lungs and brought comfort and peace.

Little by little, tension grew between Clara and me, and slowly but surely I realised that my body wasn't coping. Clara was withdrawing and we talked about my return to New Zealand. Clara had built a life of her own and I didn't fit there any longer.

I knew in my heart our relationship was ending.

Heartbreak

We were camping together at a small lake on the outskirts of Berlin. It was a warm, gentle summer night and we had spent most of it sitting together, looking into each other's eyes, seeing so much love there. I said, 'You know I have to go.'

Clara's eyes teared up. An hour later, she left the tent for a short walk. It was around one in the morning. She didn't return for some time. I began to worry so went out to find her. Approaching the lake, I heard heart-wrenching howls. Clara was sitting at the end of the jetty, crying into the starlit night. Her cries were like a wolf's, loud and echoing in the silent dark.

We both knew we had to let each other go. I sat down beside her, held her tight and we cried together.

Seemingly from nowhere, lightning pierced the darkness. Rain and wind arose with a suddenness that was frightening in intensity yet beautiful, reflecting the raw strength of our emotions. The wind swept down on us, lightning lit up the lake, thunder resounded among the hills and rain fell like our own tears.

I held Clara. Exhausted, she wept silently.

The storm passed as quickly as it had come, and the night was still again. The lake and the darkness reflected our deep love and sadness.

I had no regrets about going to Berlin to be with Clara. I tried hard. Accepting that I was not well enough to stay was a fight in itself. Clara had changed and this assured me it was our time to part. She had her life here, and mine was in New Zealand. I needed more time to heal. I had taken on too much, returning to Germany.

I was losing my best friend. I'd be alone again.

Grateful for the time I had spent in Germany with Clara, I also had a deep connection with her family, and I was glad to be able to say goodbye from the heart, face to face. One highlight was meeting Clara's grandfather who was in the Hitler youth during the Nazi regime. He fought on the front line against the Russians, then was captured and put into a Russian prison camp. He was a very clever, intelligent man and became one of the prison camp leaders. Once the war was over he made a vow to bring peace to the world. He created a political party, spoke all over the world at prestigious universities like Harvard and wrote over 100 books. I was in awe of such a man. He was now in his 90s but had a very clear mind about his past. I hung onto every word he said, sitting in his office for some hours. But what he was most proud of after all of his accomplishments and suffering was his love for his family. How proud he was of his children and great grandchildren. Love was the most important, he said in his firm yet calming German accent. 'I love my family very dearly.' The way he spoke about love touched me deeply. It's the only thing I held onto when I was in hospital.

After seven months, I flew back to New Zealand, single and sad. I had been part of a beautiful love. Now my heartache was deep. Every time it hurt, I told myself, 'You're living life fully, Josh. This sadness is good because you loved so much.'

Back home

Early October 2015. I returned home full of a sadness so deep it swallowed me whole. I was tired and desperate. I cried more than I ever did in hospital with all the shit I'd endured. This pain was different. It felt like my heart was broken in two. My whole body ached. I took my sadness and frustration and did the only thing I knew to do. I punished myself at the gym. I pushed hard, venting every emotion I had with the weight in my hand, wanting to feel the 'good' pain in every workout, feel the sweat run down my face. The more sweat I poured out, the greater my belief that my inner emotions were pouring out too. I was pushing far too hard because I wanted to feel good. Exercise had always been my friend, my release. If I'd had a bad day at work, I'd run and feel better.

I was lost, confused and hard to talk to, often asking myself what all this fight was for. I'd fought hard for love, but what was the point of that if I couldn't be with Clara?

I walked around in the deepest sadness I'd known. My head was down. My friend the wind couldn't console me. I no longer listened to the leaves falling and the trees rustling. I felt dead inside and believed that cancer should have taken me. I wanted to stop fighting and end my life. I'd been here before and knew I didn't have it in me to take my own life. However, the dark side said, 'Go on. This is the thing to do.'

It was a battle. I sat up in the Greymouth bush and cried. 'What the fuck is this all about? Why do you keep fighting, Josh? Why don't you give up, you stubborn prick?' I raged to no one.

I often asked God, 'Why are you doing this to me? Are you still with me?' I prayed, pleading, tearful, wanting to know the purpose behind this pain.

Bobby's words were always there. 'Fight 'til we get the job done.'

And Klaus's words rang in my head: 'Stay alive.'

Exercise was the only way I knew to get my mind back on track, to become fit, strong and able to run fast again. I also knew I had to talk. I remembered my psychiatrist David Garb. It was several weeks before I could bring myself to contact him. I'd been through too much and no one would understand. How could they? My whole belief in love was gone. I no longer loved myself. I'd been stripped naked and thrown into the gutter and I would not beg for help. I hated help. I hated everything, the world, my fucked-up life.

I did take comfort from my family. When extreme sadness came, my family was there. My sister Rachael was living in Brisbane, Australia with her partner Sam Thwaites. I called her and she listened patiently and cried with me. And Mum was always there, crying with me and picking me up, her hand holding mine, offering the warmth of her unconditional love. My family hugged and cried with me, they listened and it was painful for them to see their son and brother in such a state.

When I was ready, I turned to David again. We talked, laughed, and it helped. We spoke about love, whether I would ever find it again, and if anyone could love the person I had become. Clara had seen it all; she understood. Would someone else ever be as understanding?

I felt such despair because I believed I'd never find anyone, with a past and a present that were too much for a person to take on. David assured me I would, and it would be a different love.

'Keep your heart open, Josh,' he said, 'and you'll find someone.'

Even though I was distraught, David assured me those were good feelings to have. 'This is life,' he said. 'What we feel means we're living a full life, experiencing every emotion it is possible to have. It will only make you stronger, Josh.'

Talking helped and I knew that time would heal my broken heart.

I set aside thoughts of a new partner and established goals, concentrating on what I needed for myself so I could climb up and out of the dark hole. I wanted to get stronger, have the recovery I desperately needed and deserved, and leave my heart open for someone when the time was right.

Nature was calling again. My resolution for the start of 2016 was to tramp to the world's clearest lake, Blue Lake, in the Nelson Lakes National Park. I'd looked at pictures and wanted to go. Getting there would be my 'mini Everest'. I wanted to be at the lake for the dawn of the new year, to make a fresh start, swim in the lake on New Year's Day, to cleanse myself and wash away all the pain and sadness.

That was the idea anyway. I was familiar with the saying, 'The best-laid plans of mice and men go oft awry' and how life can take a totally different direction than planned. All I could do was give it a go, and if things went 'awry', my route would change too.

The walk from sadness to pain

Throughout the months leading up to the tramp, I experienced severe, nightly muscle cramps, different to those I'd had when playing sport or while training intensively. The cramps were like seizures, moving from my hips downwards as my lower body locked up.

I increased my dose of magnesium to no avail. I often woke at night with the muscles in my lower body convulsing, like waves coming onto the beach. I breathed my way through it, stretching in different positions. Sometimes I screamed and cursed aloud because the pain was so intense. There was no way I could sleep. I could only breathe, cry and try to stretch out my body. My flexibility and mobility were declining. This made me more determined to reach Blue Lake. I was not backing down.

I pushed myself at the gym, ate well, and believed my body would grow stronger and that the feelings of sadness would go. Adventure excited and motivated me. The Blue Lake was my way forward. I wanted to cleanse myself in the world's clearest water and go forward a new man, washed and healed.

The New Year was looming and it was time to go. Was I ready? I thought so. I packed my bag and drove up to St Arnaud. I planned to stay there overnight and leave for Blue Lake where I'd arranged to meet friends, Hamish and Amy. I arrived in the evening and parked at Lake Rotoiti for dinner. I sat in my deck chair by the lake and took a photo of what is probably the most photographed jetty in the world. I ate my bacon and egg pie, enjoying the stillness and the cool mountain air on my face, and thought, 'Next year is going to be a great year.' I kept repeating this in my head. It was meditative, sitting there alone, telling myself, 'I'm going to be strong. I'm going to cleanse myself in the world's clearest lake.'

A lone man walked by and I waved. He returned the wave and I invited him to have some pie with me. He smiled and said with enthusiasm, 'Yeah, why not!' Jeremy was from Switzerland, a strong man, the same age as me. We had a lot in common. As a paraglider, he loved the wind too, so we sat there chatting away and watching nature's free TV show. Jeremy's enthusiasm for life was infectious and his smile made me happy. He was going to walk the day-trip loop along the top of the hills where I was planning to go. We said goodbye, all the best, and I went to sleep in my tent.

The walk

I woke to a pleasant morning and started my walk early. I planned to make the St Angelus Hut, swim in the lake, stay the night, then continue on to Blue Lake. The sun beat down and I started to sweat heavily. After about ten minutes of walking, the waist strap broke on my backpack. The strap takes the weight of the bag around the hips. With a broken strap, I was taking the weight on my shoulders and it was pulling me towards the ground.

The track zig-zagged up the hill and I had to take a break at every corner. My body wasn't coping. I was sweating excessively and my legs where wobbling under the weight of my pack. I said to myself, 'Keep walking. Get to the top, have some lunch, stretch and make it to the hut.' I continued on.

My legs started locking up, vibrating from my bum right through to my toes. I made it to the top where a little hut was perched on the ridge. I sat down, ate my lunch and took some magnesium, salt and baking soda. I was well prepared for cramps as my legs had been seizing up frequently over the past month.

I felt a little better, spent a few more moments enjoying the beauty all around, then took up my pack and set off for the next hut where I planned to spend the night. I'd walked about 150 metres when my entire lower body locked up. My muscles in my legs convulsed up and down. The pain was intense. I yelled out aloud: "Fuuuuck!" My skinny legs were like two ice block sticks, stuck and frozen as the waves ran through the muscles. I tried to stretch but the more I moved, the worse the pain became. I lay in the tussock with my backpack on, trying to breathe through it, pleading for the pain to pass.

I tried walking again but after ten metres I was back on my arse with my legs locking up and the waves running up and down them. I lay in the tussock for what seemed hours. I looked up at the sky and screamed, 'Why the fuck can't I get a break? Why does it have to be so hard? Fuck this! I'm a loser, pathetic, useless, worthless!' I cried with sheer frustration and heartbreak, knowing I wasn't going to achieve my goal. 'Fucking cancer!' I yelled. 'Fucking transplant! Fucking life, I hate it!'

I loathed my stupid, weak body. I'd climbed to Base Camp, used to run 25 km with ease on steep terrain and now I couldn't get myself up a little hill. I was moping on my back like a frozen sheep, unable to move with the pain, crying tears like a storm. There was no way I would make it to Angelus Hut.

I had to get up and walk down the hill to the small hut where I'd had lunch. I pulled myself together. My body might've given up but my mind had not. I focused on getting there because I couldn't stay here in the scrub. I needed shelter in case the weather came in. I crawled to the hut in excruciating pain, talking to myself all the way.

I perched in the hut and drank the rest of my water, ate more food, downed a heap of electrolytes, magnesium, salt and more baking soda. My plan was to sit and wait for a few hours, then try to get the rest of the way down the hill.

A few hours passed and my legs were still not cooperating. I was feeling desperate and thought of leaving my pack, trying to get down that way, when all of a sudden Jeremy walked into the hut. I could not believe it. I was so happy and relieved to see him. His friendly smile soon turned to a look of concern.

I described my situation and he said, 'Give me your pack and I'll take you down.'

'Are you sure, bro?' I asked.

'Yeah, man. Of course, no problem.'

Off we went with my pack on one of Jeremy's shoulders and me on the other. I could walk in a few places but Jeremy insisted on helping, carrying me when I couldn't handle it. Slowly but surely we got back to the car park. He drove my car down the hill and I jumped into the lake to bathe my fatigued body. I lay in the cold water, exhausted, embarrassed and deeply hurt. I had failed to reach the Blue Lake.

I took Jeremy out for dinner as a 'thank you for saving me'. I told him everything, all about my past. He listened with empathy, not butting in or saying, 'I'm so sorry.' When I was finished he said, 'My father passed away from cancer. I've seen how tough it can be.'

I called Hamish and Amy that night, crying down the phone, so disappointed and angry. They were such great mates, understood, and said they'd be there in the morning.

I'd failed to achieve my goal and was carried out of the Blue Lake trek by a man I'd only known for 24 hours. I hated myself, my failure, my life. Being alone hurt the most. Life without Clara still cut deep. I cried myself to sleep that night.

What now . . . shingles?

Seeing my friends the next day put a smile back on my face. We headed to Hanmer Springs and stayed beside a lake. I got my swim, although it wasn't the same. Hamish and Amy helped me get back on my feet and we drove to Greymouth where I slept for a good 14 hours.

My mate Ben Wallace called to see how my New Year had gone. I told him what had happened and he invited me down to Wanaka for a few days. I jumped into the car and took off.

Wanaka is a beautiful town. The hills and the lake are so accessible. We swam and I took deep breaths of the fresh air. It was a relief to be able to tell him about my break-up with Clara, my sadness and the constant pain I felt in my skin, muscles and entire body. I left Ben's place much happier because he was a good friend trying to help as much as he could.

With my mind a bit more at ease I drove home to Greymouth to assess what I'd do for the year. I was feeling positive about my enrolment in the New Zealand Institute of Sport in Christchurch, aiming to do something productive for myself and become a personal trainer.

As I drove, I thought about my physical problems, particularly the muscle pain and the way my skin was tightening up my body. My flexibility was declining and my shoulders were becoming 'glued' into the sockets. I decided to check in with my doctor. I also felt a tickle in a tooth on the left side that extended up my cheek so figured I should add the dentist to the list.

Back home, I visited the dentist and they capped a tooth and sent me on my way.

Two days later I woke with the left side of my face swollen and tingling constantly. I went to the Greymouth hospital to find out what was wrong, confident it wouldn't be serious, that they'd give me some pills and I'd be on my way. The doctors suspected shingles so they admitted me and started IV antibiotics.

Shingles, what a joke. Just another virus the GVHD made me more susceptible to. I was disappointed but still okay with it, thinking I'd be in for a couple of nights then back home. I should have known better. It was always extreme with me, never straightforward. The next morning the left side of my face looked sunburned, bright red, scabby, swollen and worsening by the minute. I looked like Frankenstein's monster.

I had this overwhelming sense of failure. Clara, the girl I'd fought for and loved so much, had broken up with me. I had no one special to take this pain away, to hold my hand, kiss me on the forehead and say, 'I'm here, it's okay, Josh'. I'd failed my Blue Lake walk. My youth had been taken away. I wanted to be running and skydiving, not lying in this fucking bed in hospital, looking like death. I hated myself and my life. I cried and cried. Anger built up and frustration turned to desperation.

I wanted my cancer back. I wanted it to kill me because I was too scared to kill myself. I wanted an excuse to leave my fucked-up life and this madness I had created. I was falling apart. My mind was on the rampage yet again. 'When is this going to end? Can't you do anything right, Josh? No wonder Clara left you. You're a fucking loser.'

Negativity sets in so quick, and soon I was crying hysterically, thinking the cancer was back. Dad visited and I said to him, 'No more chemo, Dad. I'm going to die.' He accepted my decision and indeed I was hoping I would die. I was back in hospital, hating it. No Clara, no life, nothing.

My face got worse. It looked like someone had taken a match to it and burned my skin. I'd had enough. I pulled out the IV line, swore at the doctor and told him to kill me. I disagreed with the shingles diagnosis, convinced that the cancer was back.

'Take me to Christchurch Hospital,' I shouted. 'I hate this place. I want to be where the nurses know me and the doctors know my history.'

I wanted clarification. Was the cancer back? If so, I wanted to die where I'd started. Angry and exhausted, I rode in the ambulance for three hours to Christchurch, back to the hospital, the Bone Marrow Unit, to my familiar, safe place and the people I knew.

I was immediately at ease and more comfortable. Charge nurse Nic came in straight away and hugged me like a second mum. She asked what was wrong.

'They say it's shingles,' I said, grumpily, 'but I think my cancer's back because the left side of my face swelled up the first time I was diagnosed.'

'Don't be so sure it's cancer,' she said.

Tests and blood work showed no cancer, just a virus. Even so, my mind and outlook were black. I wanted to die because I'd had enough of hospitals and enough of pain. I felt alone. Death was the only thing that could bring me peace. If cancer returned, I could hold my mum's hand and pass away peacefully in the hospital bed where I started my journey, looking out to my tree in the park, closing my eyes, imagining I was the wind. It sounded easy.

But deep down I had more love to give, more life to live, and I tried my utmost to hold on to any glimmers of brightness.

Pain

My first night back in the Unit I woke up with a pain I could not fathom. It felt like being stabbed in the face, over and over. I screamed as I'd never screamed before, tears flooding down my cheeks. The ten minutes before it subsided felt worse than dying. I'd had no idea a person could experience or endure such pain.

'What the fuck was that?' I asked.

'That' was post-herpetic neuralgia or trigeminal neuralgia, a chronic pain affecting the trigeminal nerve, nicknamed 'the suicide disease' because about a quarter of people diagnosed with it kill themselves. After those few minutes with it, I could understand why. For six weeks I was hooked up to morphine while my face burned and the nerve itself vibrated under the skin, its pulses running up and down like an electric current, keeping me tensed for the next explosion.

The second jolt of pain came after about three hours. It was too much. I needed Mum, Clara, someone, anyone, to hold my hand. I'd always been able to focus my mind and control pain to some degree, but not for this. After the second time I called Mum. Once again, her understanding workplace gave her leave. She was there to hold my hand.

Another attack came, then another, torture after torture. I tried to hold onto visions of myself doing the things I loved, happy, free, in love with a beautiful woman, but I was so scared of the pain, terrified like a little boy.

The worst occurred at 11 one night. A 15-minute attack. Both nurses were there holding my hands. They gave me as much pain relief as possible, but nothing worked. I was screaming, begging them to kill me, pleading with God to stop the pain. I opened my eyes for one second and Courtney, one of the nurses, was crying because she could do nothing more for me. I was sent to ICU to have lignocaine to help numb the nerve. I had three infusions into my blood stream, through a 'pick' line, every second day for a week.

The pain went on.

I prayed to God. Every half hour, sometimes every minute, I pictured a simple life, with love and health. And so I wrote:

That's all I want. It's not much, is it? I'm in love with someone, I'm healthy, I'm happy and I'll fight for ten minutes of that pure love. God wouldn't let me suffer for no reason. He chose me for something. I'm different. I'm Josh Komen. I'll do everything I can to survive even though the days get tough, dark and scary. I'll continue on, I'll pursue to the end. I hate this pain, but love who I am.

Suffering builds and moulds you into a better you, but only if you're willing. I'm still grateful to be who I am.

I'd kept a pain diary since the first diagnosis. Writing gave me an outlet to spill my thoughts, a way to vent frustration, anger and pain. It enabled me to express feelings when I couldn't give voice to them. I spoke with my hand, pen on paper, and the words spoke back to me, helping me push on and endure.

I started to write about the shingles, my weak body and shit life. I wrote with anger and frustration, and yet with deep gratitude for all I had achieved. I gripped that pen tight.

From the pain diary

I needed someone to hold my hand.

After that agony I wanted someone to be there for me, hold my hand, squeeze it tight. I didn't want to be alone. I was scared.

When I was first diagnosed, I didn't want anyone around. Stubborn.

Now I just wanted a hand to hold.

Mum came. She was there.

A spider web under my face.

In the middle it burns like a house on fire. My firemen struggle to contain the fire. The web is long, thick and tight, it extends to the drill hole in my head. The firemen hold position. If the fire comes up the web, if the firemen can't contain it, the drill drills into my brain, then the grater starts up behind my eye, the web ignites into raging flames. The knife sticks in and runs up and down my face while the drill is still drilling, the grater is grating the back of my eye, the knife is slashing, the fire burning.

I'm screaming, yelling.

The water comes to wash away everything but sometimes it doesn't work. Sometimes the web wins. The web is always there, the firemen are always fighting. I am fighting. This is real pain. This is fighting. This is surviving.

I'm too scared to scratch my head or touch my face because the pain will come.

This drug ketamine (*used for sedation and pain relief*)

makes you someone else. I'm struggling to be me on the outside. I picture running through a field, long grass, bare feet, hands by my sides. The sun shines bright upon my face, a field of green, a sky of blue, fresh clean air, a smell I can't describe.

I'm free.

I run with a smile. A light drizzle starts. I take my clothes off and feel the rain. I lie in the grass, naked as the day I was born. The rain cleanses me. It feels so good. The sun fights through the clouds, dries my wet body. I lie there with a smile that no one can take away, happy, free.

9.30 pm 24 January 2016

Worst pain of my life.

Please, God, take this away. The pain has not stopped. It's been back to back, unreal. I didn't think it possible. My painful life.

5.30 pm 25 January 2016

Today's pain is something else. I can't describe it.

I never knew there was such pain, left side of my face, constant tremors telling me it's there. It is so scary.

My heart rate is around 130–140. I'm so anxious. I don't want the pain to come. I pray and pray, ask for forgiveness, ask why, ask God to heal me. I know He will. I trust God. I do.

26 January 2016

My face is burning. I'm glad it's not my head. It's sore but bearable, like little ants or spiders running under my skin with flames.

I hate the position I'm in. Fuck my body. Why has God let this happen? Fuck, this is tough. I cannot believe I'm going through all this pain.

I'm containing the pain in my face. I sit in bed, alone, no

one next to me. How has this happened? I want this to end.

My eyes shut, then open. What is happening? Am I dying? The pain tells me I'm still alive. It knocks its sharp hand on my face. Fuck off. Give me peace. I've had enough.

My face burns. I've never felt like this. Is it my time?

Ruth called. We talked, laughed and cried. She's a real friend. Thank you, Ruth, from the bottom of my heart.

Please God, I pray for peace.

I can't believe the pain. I want to die but want to live. I have so much to give. If I die I want to be with God. If I live, God, please bless me.

Am I giving up?

The pain medication has turned me in to a zombie. I speak mumbled gibberish.

I don't know where, or who, I am.

People visit but I don't want them here for long in case I have an attack. I don't want them to see me screaming, crying, shouting out, Kill me!

It's a minute-by-minute battle. The pain overwhelms me and I want to die, truly, I do. I tell Mum every day to kill me, please kill me. No mother should have to experience this. She called David Garb and he came in to talk.

Together, David and I decided that there was still a lot of good in my life and, deep down, I wanted to live. It was this sheer torment in my face, this pain, that I wanted to have die, not me, so I fought on, praying the pain would go, asking God every second to help me. My faith grew much stronger.

The pain told me I wanted to die. I told the pain I was alive. I held on to the inner love I felt for myself, my love of nature, for Mum and my friends.

I've taken a lot of pain over these years, all kinds of pain – physically and mentally. Why don't I just give up?

I want to some days but it's just not in me any more to do that, no matter how tough it gets.

I've asked Dad, Mum, the nurses, to kill me because I'm in so much pain, but maybe I'm just saying that in the moment. Once it's gone, I'm fine. Once you get the worst of it, like last night, three times in such a short stint, you say, well, it can't get much worse than that.

I love my family too, so much – Mum, Dad, Rach and Jake. They are so amazing. I fight for the plain simplicity of loving someone. Being in love, doing the thing I love. Just being normal.

Day by day I do little things: rest, read and write when I can, eat when I'm able to, think of my next move, picture myself fit and healthy and in love.

I want this to end so bad. I ring Dad and Mum and I cry. I have to hold on.

My body scares me. I used to love it but it scares me so much. Every tingle, every sensation scares the fuck out of me. I flinch. Please ease this pain. Please go away.

I want a good night's sleep, a good 24 hours with no pain.

Push on, Josh, push forward. You're not alone.

I wish Clara was here holding my hand though she wouldn't like to see this.

I feel like a pin cushion. They struggle to get blood due to my thick skin. I'm not kidding. Over these last three weeks they've tried to get needles in at least 30 times. I just lay my arm out and say, 'Do it.' That pain is nothing compared to what I've been having.

They've changed the drug to ketamine with fentanyl. I pray it helps, just to get some peace.

My face is so sore. 24/7 little bugs run up and down my skin, telling me, Josh, we're here and we're going to fuck you up.

10.33 pm – I don't know what day it is
Please, God, take this pain away. This is all I ask. A man can only take so much.

Do I want to die? Yes, then no.

It feels like the German army is running up and down my face. Let me out of here.

I talked to Clara. I can tell she doesn't even want to be friends. She doesn't seem to care.

She has a new friend. She has changed. Her attitude, her words were nothing and didn't help. I fell in love with the wrong girl. Can someone change so quickly?

Things are different and I need to move on. I have the wisdom to know that, but in my heart I'll always love her. She'll always be a part of me. I'll write one final letter to her.

She broke my heart.

Josh, go forward with wisdom and common sense. You've got to keep your head up. Keep going, Josh.

Nurses, doctors, orderlies, hospital

How grateful I am to have these people around in my time of need. I'm drugged off my head right now after such a painful day and there's more to come. Lidocaine, fentanyl, ketamine, nortriptyline, tramadol, gabapentin. It reads like a pharmaceutical dictionary. Everyone is trying and so am I because I want this gone, to live my life, be free.

Thank you, nurses, doctors, people who have helped. Angels on feet with no wings, but arms – thank you for the hands to hold.

I do hope this new drug regime will help. I pray for no more pain. I want out so bad, but will be patient and finish this job.

27 January 2016

I had one attack today but it didn't last as long.

The pain sits in the background all the time, like a spider web over my face. The spiders are like fire, running up and down. I have a drill hole above my head. When the pain ignites, the web tightens and grows, the spiders start to crawl and when the web hits the drill hole the volcano of pain erupts. I still feel the pain, but the drugs I'm on now lower the intensity.

I picture firemen with cold foam spraying the web and the spiders.

The firemen fight and then I picture my nerves getting cleaned with a paint brush so they're brand new, even better than before, everything is okay and there will be no long-term damage.

I hope it continues to work because they've done all they can.

The medication messes me up physically. Although my speech is bad, my mind is clear. I can think and listen, picture myself where I need to be, see what I need to do. They say this can last up to three months. So far it's been three and a bit weeks. I ask God why He let this happen.

Mostly I pray to God to either kill me, or get me through this, to heal and bless me.

I have great nurses. Courtney is amazing. When I'm in pain, she puts the fentanyl in and holds my hand. I like this a lot.

30 January 2016

Constant pain in my face but no attacks overnight.

Nurses let me sleep until 10 am. Awesome! Things are feeling better. The firemen are putting out the fire. My face feels like a lump of clay.

I push the pain button (*to release IV medication*) often though because the fire is always there.

I want to use my mind to fight it but the doctors and nurses insist I use the button, so I am, although it is my choice. They check how many times I use it.

Coming down the mountain. A couple of steep bits in between, painful but tolerable. Push the green button for relief.

Beautiful day outside. I want to be out there, on my slackline, balancing and breathing as I walk the line. Swimming, laughing, sharing the day with friends.

How I'd love to be healthy, to run and win a race, just one. Become a physiotherapist, explore New Zealand, learn, grow, pray, heal, inspire, show people how to never give up.

Please, God, heal my face.

1 February 2016

I am living a full life, feeling everything possible: pain, love, hate.

Hate is the same as love, just a flip of the coin, because one cannot live without the other.

I feel all that is around me without opening my eyes. I appreciate the green leaves blowing, the grass growing, bit by bit. I choose to take the good. I choose to love. I feel everything.

I am a child, longing inside for the simple things that fulfil me. I have loved and lost, I have laughed and cried.

Pain is going. No attacks now for nearly three days.

11.12 pm. I now call it a Drill Pain. It burns and stings and I get Drill attacks. The nurses let me sleep. They took blood and I didn't even wake up. I need sleep.

Keep stretching, keep writing, keep focusing, Josh, you're winning.

2 February 2016

Off the ketamine although the fire burns constantly in my face. It hurts and I often push the green button. I'm getting physio too. That's good.

I'm shaking, pushing the green button. I'd love not to feel anything on my face. I'm so tired. You can see it in my eyes.

I watch the runners go past.

This is the best I've felt all month. I've fought, I've prayed.

I thank God for where I am now. I'm excited for the future. I've changed.

Something has happened to me. My faith in God is stronger than ever. My face is still sore but I'm happy where I am.

The tide is turning. I'm growing stronger inside myself. There are amazing people in my life. I'm experiencing everything.

I wipe my tears. The sun rises. Tomorrow is another day.

Brian Bell. What a man. How blessed I am to have him in my life. We prayed together which was nice. We talked and laughed. Thanks, Brian. It was an absolute pleasure to have you here. What a friend.

Send me an angel

Please, God, send me an angel, an angel to protect and free me from this pain, someone to hold my hand.

I see myself walking hand in hand along the beach with a beautiful girl. It's a summer day. A gentle wind blows, I hear the sound of the ocean on the sand and against the rocks.

I'm in love. We've both suffered but we're free for this moment. I feel the wind wrap around me, I know God has blessed me. I come home to my beautiful wife – we smile at how blessed we are. We love and care for people, for each other.

We look into each other's eyes and appreciate what we have and the love we share. I can't have kids though I do picture them running, laughing in front of us. Maybe I can have kids. I'll care for them utterly, unconditionally. I am at peace.

We have kids, a garden, live by the ocean. We welcome everyone, cook healthy, tasty meals.

God is watching over us. No pain.

Just peace and love. No pain.

No pain.

Skydiving

I long for the freedom. The door opens, the wind hits my face, I'm truly alive.

I'm jumping from 12,000 feet. Are you mad?

I'm living, falling fast, looking and smiling at my friends. How blessed I am. I pull my pilot chute, it opens full and I float. I'm in control. I love this, my favourite part. No rules, find my landing spot, how blessed I am to be doing this.

Naked in the rain

I wish I was standing in the rain, naked, hands in the sky, feeling the rain. It's a warm day. The rain hits my body. It cleanses me. It's beautiful.

The sun in my pocket

The pain was now somewhat under control, though the left side of my face burned as if it was on fire. I was allowed to go outside when things had stabilised, and breathe the fresh air I longed for. An orderly took me out, and once in nature I grabbed the sun and put it in my pocket, embracing the world and pulling it into my soul, holding onto mother nature like a new-found lover. Back in my room I let out the sun in small pieces, pretending it was shining on me. That brought me happiness and joy. I laughed at my childlike self, but no one was around to judge me.

Little things got me through the days. I remembered the feel of the wind hitting my face like a cold blanket. I visualised the warmth of the sun, shining as brightly as the love from my beautiful, graceful Mum.

I worked at taking my frustration, pain and anger away to some happy space, but it was hard. Clara had been happiness, but she was gone, so I was left with my own thoughts. I remembered the Coast Road, my hometown, skydiving, all of the things I longed to do for myself. I wanted to find a new girlfriend, someone special.

I was lost, lonely and came closer to God. Reading the Bible gave me strength, as did the visits from my friends and family. One visitor in particular gave me so much when I needed it most. When I was growing up, my neighbor Adam 'Neukes' Newcombe was my idol. He was the man in my world who taught me how to shoot a basketball, kick-flip a skateboard and to get on with girls. Adam was diagnosed with prostate cancer a year before I was in hospital with the pain. We grew close. On this visit we talked about the hardship cancer brings, how fatigued and exhausted we were. How it affects not only us, but our families, not to mention our finances. Losing your job and having a limited income restricts what you can and cannot do, and cancer also burdens those close to you. Normal life has been taken away – from the people we love too. We talked deep and encouraged each other. Together we could laugh about how the drinking water on our street must have been contaminated with cancer. We talked about his little girl Willow and his wife Anna, how much he loved them. We talked about the special people in our lives who helped us on the journey.

I read through the pages of my pain diary and admired my own strength to carry on. My mum never cried in front of me. She sat silently and held my hand tight. Mum was brave, far braver than me as I screamed like a child for her to kill me. If the knife piercing my skull had been real, there were times when I would have turned it on myself. My mum, and the visualisations I held within, gave me the determination not to give up.

Can you please wash higher?

Despite the pain and the tears of this fucked-up situation, there were times I could see the funny side. In intensive care, where I was getting lignocaine infusions, a support nurse came and asked if I'd like a bed bath.

'Yes please,' I moaned.

The nurse was about 60. I hadn't washed in a long time, and

with the constant sweat running down my body I wasn't smelling too good.

She brought over a bucket of hot soapy water and a sponge and began washing my legs and inner thighs. I felt something I hadn't experienced in months. I was getting aroused. Even drugged off my head I still felt the tingling sensation run through my body.

I grinned and asked the nurse, 'Can you please wash higher?' She laughed and said, 'No, sorry, love. It's just the legs today,' and we both had a chuckle.

I rested my head on the pillow and enjoyed the warm soapy sponge running up and down my legs.

If it's not pain . . . it's GVHD

After two months in the Bone Marrow Unit, screaming, crying and being depressed, the pain was under control. The left side of my face was numb and I was told I might not get any feeling back. Our concern moved to the GVHD, which had worsened since Jeremy carried me off the hill at Lake Rotoiti.

GVHD is a cruel disease. I became the Tin Man, stiff as a brick. My muscles were gluing together. I could only get my hands to above my knees and had painful cramp seizures in my legs. I couldn't lift my arms above my head. I was stuck, sore and weak.

GVHD can attack any organ in the body. For some reason it had chosen my skin, muscles, fascia, tendons and ligaments. The name of this new disease was chronic graft versus host disease scleroderma, a thickening of the skin. The build-up of a protein called collagen glued my body together and the pigmentation in my skin was disappearing. It was so painful and sucked life from within.

My body was constantly fighting to the point of sheer exhaustion and I looked like an old man. I couldn't produce saliva and my eyes where always blood shot and dry. My body had become so tight I couldn't put my socks on and I struggled to bend over and pick up objects from the ground. My abdominals cramped and locked every time I bent forward, my legs would spasm uncontrollably, my skin was dry, sore and red, and my shoulders where glued in place like small branches hanging off a tree. I couldn't lift them up. I was in 24-hour pain. The disease is treatable, though the high dose medication is not fun. Doses of both the steroids and cyclosporine (an immune suppressant) were increased. Dr Ganly was concerned and knew something had to be done.

I returned to Greymouth at the start of March 2016, after a torturous couple of months, my face still burning, my body stuck together and my mind scrambled, weak and exhausted. I had to go back to square one and start healing all over again.

I did my yoga (though it might not have looked like your yoga) and a lot of basic exercises, morning and night, to maintain what stamina and flexibility I still had. I spent a lot of time with my masseuse, my good friend Dave Gordon who gave me a massage twice a week. He had helped me a lot when I was running and now the goal was to maintain the limited movement I still had. Though I was on a high dosage of steroids and immuno suppressant drugs the GVHD was slowly taking over and more action needed to be taken.

Dr Ganly and Dr Ruth Spearing advocated for me to receive Extracorporeal Photopheresis (ECP) treatment at the Peter MacCallum Cancer Centre in Melbourne, Australia. Peter Mac is a leading cancer research, treatment and education centre, and Australia's only public hospital dedicated to treating people affected by cancer. The treatment wasn't available in New Zealand, but a handful of Kiwis were receiving the treatment for GVHD and getting good results, especially with skin and muscles.

The treatment and accommodation were fully funded. All I had to do was buy my own food.

I'd researched the holistic approach to healing and the mind-body connection, seen several practitioners and never really clicked with any of them, as I needed to hear a scientific explanation. The words 'because it's good for you' just didn't cut it. Some of the doctors called these ideas hocus-pocus, but I'd come to believe that alternative therapies and ideas had a place, integrated with modern medicine to achieve the best possible outcome.

I didn't believe in monotherapy, a one-fix wonder. I incorporated many different tools, such as exercise, food and meditation to get the best quality of life possible. I had previously completed a certificate in nutrition so I could gain a better understanding of food and make more informed choices. However, I knew I also needed someone I could relate to, who understood me, to help me through my treatment and recovery. I was always looking for alternative answers. I was very grateful and keen to try the treatment offered in Melbourne. I had high hopes it would change or even reverse the GVHD and restore some quality of life.

Most of all, I hoped it could take away the pain I constantly lived with.

Melbourne is waiting

I had one month to regain some strength so while at home on the Coast, I breathed in the fresh air, ate and rested well. I used visualisations constantly, did yoga, prayed to God, which all had a positive effect for me.

I ate as well as I could and experimented with a few different diets. I'd stopped drinking long ago. My battle so far had been extreme. I'd learned so much about the human body, what can and cannot be of benefit, and I was still looking for significant help, physically and mentally.

Melbourne was waiting and I hoped it would provide more medical and holistic healing opportunities. I'd spoken to a lady Ellen Minchin who was just finishing her treatment in Melbourne, the treatment that I'd be getting. Ellen said it was exhausting and tiring but nothing like chemo. That was a relief to hear.

I focused on how amazing I'd feel after this treatment, picturing myself running, skydiving and climbing a mountain again, helping others, falling in love, praying and loving God. I'd never give up.

I'd suffer, push, cry, laugh, feel the wind and fight. I would survive.

I was to live in Melbourne for six months while I received treatment, initially three times a week. Then it would reduce to twice a week for three months, followed by twice every fortnight. When the treatment became monthly I would fly back and forth.

My Melbourne apartment was in The Quest building, right in the heart of the city on Lonsdale Street, not far from Peter Mac. A yoga centre was nearby and my friends Dave Ridley, Paddy Nichols, Josh McEwen and Jase Jacobs lived there too, so I'd have some company during my stay.

People said, 'Wow, Melbourne, that's a cool holiday!' It was going to be no vacation. I enjoy cities and all they offer but after a while, I feel like a rat in a cage, longing for nature, peace and quiet. The job was to get better, and hopefully find someone, something to help and guide me alongside my treatment.

I arrived in Melbourne on 1 April 2016, exhausted from the flight. Jacob, my brother, travelled with me which was comforting since he was my best mate. I was so grateful to have him by my side, helping me every way he could. Once we landed in Melbourne I collapsed outside the airport, exhausted from the flight and the procedure done in Christchurch Hospital two days beforehand: having a new Hickman line inserted into my chest. Jake called a taxi, which took us to The Quest.

My apartment was small and reminded me of those East Berlin apartment units, empty and dark. However, the accommodation gave me the freedom to cook, shower, sleep and do yoga. It was enough. I knew I could be somewhere far worse.

The city was loud, chaotic, full-on, cold and wet. The sun went down fast in the winter. I was still weak from all the pain and medications of the previous months. I'd hit the wall hard. I'd never experienced fatigue like it, even after working 12 hard physical hours cutting a load of firewood, followed by a 16 km run. That is a 'good' tired. This was an exhaustion that I lost myself in. My whole body collapsed. I felt my eyes roll back in my head. I had bricks on my eyebrows and the weight of ten men pulling me down to the earth.

Jake stayed with me for the first two weeks, helping me to set up. I was glad he was there. One day I went exploring in the city by myself and while waiting for a tram my whole body locked up. My legs were stuck and I spent two hours rolling around uncontrollably on a bench. People passing by must have thought I was a crazy man and no one stopped to ask if I was okay. I managed to phone Jacob. He came to the tram stop and helped me on my way.

My body would cramp and lock up spontaneously during the day. When I slept my feet and hips would lock up, the frequent episodes giving me torturous cramps. I'd scream out aloud as I jumped from the bed. It was hard to get enough sleep, and without it I struggled like a lost zombie the following day. This was the constant daily battle of mind over body. Sometimes I'd cry with the pain, sometimes I'd laugh. I longed for a 'normal' middle ground.

I was longing for this treatment to turn things around. I had a body, but couldn't use it properly. The mind would want do something, but the body would not follow. It was frustrating and exhausting. I wanted my independence back and some freedom from the daily pain.

After the experience at the tram stop, which was happening more frequently now, I decided to stay close to the apartment, only visiting close facilities such as the supermarket, Fitzroy Park, Peter Mac and the yoga centre. That was all I needed for now.

Peter Mac

The Peter McCallum Cancer Centre was a short walk from the apartment. I'd go there three times the first week then twice a week for the following months. My job was to get better. I read books about healing the body at the cellular level and other motivational resources, drew inspiration from yoga, meditation and visualisation, and I prayed to God.

I was excited and nervous walking into my first round of treatment.

I told myself, this is it, Josh. This is where you will heal. The treatment will reverse the GVHD. It will work.

I had ECP treatment in the Apheresis department. The team were great, less formal than the Christchurch nurses. Right away Jack was going on at me about being a Kiwi; the ice was broken and the banter flowed back and forth. The team was small: Jack, Aaron, Paige, James, Marg, and Annette who was the 'team mother'. The load on my shoulders would lighten at treatment time as I knew there would be laughter and fun.

The Hickman line that was inserted into my chest was a blessing. I wouldn't have to have the two needles that looked like nine-inch nails driven into my arms.

Extracorporeal phototheresis (ECP) involves the removal and separation of blood – about 1.5 litres – into white and red blood cells. The white cells – my immune system – were attacking my body, reading it as foreign and signalling other cells to join the attack. Once the blood had been drawn then separated into red and white blood cells, the red cells where returned back to me via the central line that drew the blood and then back into my blood stream.

The white blood cells that remained were then treated with a special serum called 'UVADEX.' This was used to target a particular diseased white blood cell called a 'T-Lymphocyte' – T-cell. The remaining white blood cells were then exposed to ultra violet light. The combination of the serum and the ultra violet light damaged the diseased T-cells causing apoptosis (cell death). The treated white cells were then returned back to me via the same central line. It was then up to my own immune system to 'up-regulate' healthy T-Lymphocytes to attack the treated dying T-Lymphocytes, which would then 'down-regulate' the Graft Vs Host Disease. It's incredible what science can do!

The procedure lasted roughly two to three hours. I felt nothing, though halfway through I'd fall asleep from the exhaustion of having so much blood removed. At the beginning and end of the treatment I managed to chat and have a laugh with other patients and the nurses.

The ECP treatment is the last outpost for patients who've had all the chemo, radiation, the transplant and now have severe GVHD. It is for 'the worst of the worst', the people who have endured heart, lung, or bone marrow transplants like me, to stop graft rejection. ECP offers the final fragment of hope for restoring the quality of life that the vampire GVHD has sucked away.

Everyone undergoing ECP hopes the treatment will reverse the rejection. The Peter Mac Apheresis team knew that and understood the suffering that brought patients to their door. They offered unconditional kindness, humour, empathy and love. They made me smile and laugh from my belly. I met other patients who'd lost their looks, their functions, nearly lost their minds too, sucked away by the vampire within. We sat in our chairs, hooked up to the machine, watching the blood being drawn from our veins and separated, praying that this would reverse the GVHD.

GVHD is not for the faint-hearted. For cancer there's the treatment that kills cancer cells and it sometimes succeeds. GVHD is persistent and there's no cure – the hope lies in treatments that suppress the immune system and help the body adjust to the 'new normal'. It's a chronic disease that deteriorates the body, changes it and can kill it. My muscles were glued up. My skin pigmentation had changed. With no saliva production, I couldn't swallow food without water. My eyes were constantly red and ached from dryness, feeling as if little metal scraps were lodged under the lids, and my legs cramped and locked up uncontrollably at any given time. Was this what life had come to? Being an old man decades before my time. Painfully stuck and exhausted. It was worse than cancer because I was alive living outside my safe little isolation room but I couldn't live as I wanted to. Simple things like putting my clothes and socks on or tying my shoes were a struggle. Walking a small distance took every ounce of effort as my body would lock up at every little motion. This wasn't the person I wanted to be.

Tracie was from Christchurch. She was receiving treatment too and stayed in the same apartment building. We became good mates, enjoyed a laugh together and often talked about how much cancer and the severe GVHD had affected our quality of life. She was in her 40s, married with two children, and arrived every month for her treatment. She would fly in for her treatment the following day and on the night of her arrival she'd come to my apartment where I cooked dinner because I knew how tired she'd be.

At the start of our treatment neither of us could produce saliva, so one evening we decided to have a spitting competition. Tracie's first spit was just a puff, nothing at all. I gave her some chocolate and she spat this dark, round, lugie into my living room. It tumbled out of her mouth, down her chin and onto the floor and we both laughed so hard. She was a hard case, that's for sure.

Yoga

I had a limited amount of money to spend in Melbourne and kept to a tight budget. I got quite good at sneaking onto the trams, sitting at the back and hopping off if I saw a guard. I shopped at the Victoria market, buying meat, fish and vegetables for less than at the supermarket. My budget allowed for one or two extra health services and yoga proved to be good value for money.

Melbourne life was tough on my own. I had to gather all my strength for the simplest tasks, plus I had to shop for groceries, cook, and get to treatment in my glued-up body. I often slept for several hours during the day, not wanting to go out into the chaotic city. I had a job to complete so I could go home. Plain and simple. I wanted my body back so I could run, swim, jump and climb and work again. I pleaded with God, praying with pure intention, to please let this treatment work.

Yoga helped and became my new routine, my 'running practice'. I was a regular at the nearby studio. A good friend sent me the link to a crazy Dutch guy who had developed his own method, 'the Wim Hof method', with scientific evidence that it decreased inflammation in the body. Wim's training combined with breathing, cold exposure, mindset techniques and physical exercises to improve health and wellbeing. When the opportunity arose to do an online ten-week course I paid my money, completed the programme and found it incredibly beneficial. The breathing was profound, consisting of thirty to forty deep breaths then holding your breath after the last round. I had an energy I hadn't felt in years; my body was tingling with excitement. After the breathing, Wim advocated a cold shower or an ice bath. I was a tad nervous heading into the cold shower but I'd had experience of it in my running days. That combined with the breathing was powerful. I felt as if I'd taken drugs! I was fully focused, alert and pain-free for several hours afterwards. This method had a profound impact on my depression as I felt empowered, ready to tackle the world, no fears, no worries. I was hooked and practised the method daily.

I can't live. I can only function

The days went by. Melbourne was so different to my Greymouth paradise. Homeless people begged on the streets. The sun went down early and the city fell into darkness. I wasn't used to that. I was alone most of the time. I craved nature and the outdoors so spent hours in Fitzroy Park, doing yoga and meditating, feeling nature all around me. I attended evening yoga classes, returned to my little apartment, cooked dinner, and fell asleep.

Every night I dreamed of my past running on the Coast Road with Ruth and Eddie, climbing a hill with Ben or simply putting on my overalls and going to work. In my waking hours, I pictured myself travelling with Jake, jumping out of the plane with Matt, Iohann and Wayne Holmes, chopping firewood with Hamish. I missed my life. It was hard to let go of a past I loved so much and I clung to these visions.

There was always pain in my legs. Every morning when I got out of bed, they would lock up and I had to breathe through the pain for 15 minutes before staggering to a cold shower. I saw an old man looking at me from the mirror, a skinny, frail person with the pigmentation disappearing from his skin. I looked completely different from who I was last year.

The cold shower worked wonders: no pain, just pure, fresh, coldness embracing me. I felt good under the cold water. However, my body ached all day and my head was foggy, as if I'd been on the piss for a week. No matter how much I slept it was always the same and I wondered what was with that? I was jealous and angry and often said to myself, 'Every other fucker can go to sleep, wake up and feel fine, but not me.' It was stupid talk, but such thoughts popped up and I had to let them go. Every day I tried so hard to make my life better, to improve my health, but then something else would come up, something new, to remind me that I can't live, I can only function and struggle like a two-year-old with this fucked-up mess of a body.

I descended to the dark place again, dwelling on all that had gone wrong and all I'd lost.

I wanted to be Physical Josh again, fit and active, the guy who could do a standing backflip, instead of this stiff old man hobbling about, weary and sad. I cried for my poor self, dwelling on the past, staggering around this city of strangers where no one knew me or cared about all I'd been through.

I wrote in my diary, shedding my pain through words, asking God why He let me suffer so. I tried to focus on the good, remembering my family, all of the people who'd come into my life since childhood and those special friends who were always there for me.

I had never backed down from a challenge but some days I wanted to let go and I figured it would be easier for everyone if I died. I still found it hard to accept this new Josh.

Alone in ICU

Since arriving in Melbourne I'd been having a pain in my chest. Some days it was a niggle that bothered me when I walked or lay down to sleep. Other days it felt like a hot poker prodding me. Sometimes I wanted to die because of the pain and then I hated myself for thinking about dying and knew I should be grateful.

Be patient, they said.

I've been like this for six years. I was still aching and not fulfilling my life. I thought of what I could achieve if my body worked properly. I'm not patient.

I was receiving treatment one day when they found a marker in my blood indicating an inflammation of the heart. I was admitted to the Peter McCallum ICU unit so they could monitor me for the night. Once again, I was alone in hospital without family or friends. In the morning, I got out of bed and collapsed with a searing pain in my chest, shaking and sweating. Ten doctors swarmed over me. They administered meds and soon I was comfortable.

I spent another two nights in the ICU. It was tough being there alone. My friends in Melbourne were working and by the end of the day I was too tired for them to visit.

My chest didn't improve and the pain progressed. The doctors were puzzled. A cardiac stress test indicated something wrong with my heart so they followed up with an angiogram. This was also inconclusive. The arteries were clear. I was discharged.

I received news from home that my good friend Adam Newcombe had passed away. I flew back to speak at his funeral. Adam left behind his beautiful girl Willow and strong, loving wife Anna. I was deeply saddened by the loss of my friend. Adam had been a role model and a comfort for me. If I could have traded my life for his, I would have. I asked God why I was still alive and Adam wasn't. I felt a deep love for this man who had befriended me, gave me laughter and the blessing of his time and attention. I thought about the good that I, too, would leave behind, and I knew I had to keep fighting.

A return to Melbourne

I went back to Melbourne and the pain in my chest continued, waking me up at night. I'd been practising the Wim Hof Method of cold showers followed by deep breathing and meditation. The Method gave me clarity of thought, increased my energy and inspired a more positive mindset. My medications were decreasing but my body was still extremely tight. I was weak and in constant pain. I pushed on, looking forward to the Wim Hof retreat I'd signed up for near Melbourne.

Hamish flew over for a visit. We watched a few rugby league games and I taught him all I had learned about the Wim Hof Method. It was a relief to have him with me. I could talk to Hamish about my feelings, about the loneliness that consumed me in such a big city and how homesick I was for Greymouth. Another good friend, Andrew Nidd, flew into Melbourne to surprise me for the weekend, and Matt and his wife Millie paid a visit too. My good friends were there, doing all they could to help.

The kindness of friends

The trigeminal neuralgia had damaged the nerves and numbed the left side of my face. The pain doctors in Christchurch Hospital told me I probably wouldn't get the feeling back. I didn't want to hear that, so started my own research, reading that hyperbaric oxygen therapy could have a beneficial effect on the nerves in the human body. I was keen to give it a try. It was expensive. I could afford a few hours but knew I'd need far more.

I came home from a small walk in Fitzroy Park one day to find that Matt and Millie had set up a Givealittle funding page to raise money for more oxygen treatment. I was surprised and overwhelmed. Tears rolled down my cheeks. During their visit I'd told them about the treatment and my hope that it might help. Thanks to the Givealittle page they set up, I was able to have 70 hours in the hyperbaric oxygen chamber.

The left side of my face is now normal and I have feeling.

The kindness of good friends is humbling. They are a true blessing.

Heartache

I continued the treatments, walking over to Peter Mac as usual. The chest was getting much worse, then one night I woke with excruciating pain. My hands were clenched against my chest and I forced myself to breathe deeply and relax as the Wim Hof Method had taught me. I was afraid of going into cardiac arrest alone in my little apartment room. I had the Hickman line in my chest for the treatment and I wondered if the line was aggravating something. After the all-clear angiogram, my Melbourne doctor Simon Harrison was thinking similarly because the pain started when the line went in at the start of April.

The doctors took the line out two days before the Wim Hof retreat. I felt somewhat better, the pain less intense. A bus took us to the retreat out on the Ocean Road. I met the other participants over dinner. All the while the pain was niggling in the background, making it hard for me to engage in conversation. I managed to sleep a few hours, wrestling with the pain. Then in the morning I awoke to the most intense pain rushing through my chest. It felt as though someone was squeezing my heart, I struggled to breathe and in my distress called for help. 'Please someone, please help, I can't get out of bed. My chest, my chest!' I moaned in despair.

A man I didn't know heard me, called an ambulance and comforted me while we waited. I later found out he was Guy Lawrence, founder of 180 Nutrition. The pain was horrible. I breathed as best I could, closed my eyes and prayed I wouldn't go into cardiac arrest. The ambulance arrived and I left the retreat without attending a single hour.

Besides the pain, I felt sadness and frustration. What was the point of setting goals? Every time I did, something else happened. Why couldn't I just enjoy myself, meet these exciting, new people, experience something I was so looking forward to? I cried hard in the ambulance. I was in a dark hole, alone and tangled up in barbed wire, every movement painful, my body stuck fast, with nothing to pull me out.

My mind was in turmoil, fighting with my past, hating my present, and here I was again, all alone, in an ambulance, no family or friends, just me, my thoughts and God. I tried to jog myself along. Come on, this was just another hurdle, I'd had worse to get over. I felt torn between wanting to live and giving up, the continual cycle. I knew how good life could be when those small perfect moments occurred, the ones that brought such joy. I hung onto them, held them close, with an unshakeable belief that I'd survive, then thrive, after all this bullshit. I was in quicksand, yes, but there was light, and I tried so hard to savour it.

Multiple heart attacks

I had one episode of chest pain after another in at Geelong Hospital. I called my sister and said I'd had enough and wanted to die. I cried and swore at the doctors because they seemed to be treating me as a number, not a person. I stayed one night at Geelong before going back to Peter McCallum in Melbourne.

I apologised for swearing. I don't think I was forgiven. They were pleased to see the back of me.

They all knew me at Peter Mac and I felt comfortable in the familiar surroundings. My Auntie Bernie flew in from Sydney. She sat with me and held my hand while I cried and had yet another heart attack. To have Bernie's hand in mine was all I needed. She gave me strength. I could see and feel the depth of her love for me.

Dr Simon Harrison witnessed my agony, seeing firsthand what I'd been trying to describe. He transferred me to the Royal Melbourne Cardiac Unit across the road. I breathed and meditated my way through the attacks, to the amazement of the doctors who couldn't understand why I was no longer swearing and crying. I lay there, did my Wim Hof breathing, slow and focused, concentrating and telling myself I was strong and I'd had far worse pain.

I was desperate for something to be done.

Mum flew over to be with me. She'd seen everything and now

had to watch her son have heart attacks. I felt for her. Mum's inner strength and love picked me up and pushed me through, comforting me in this life-threatening situation. Her strength made me stronger. If she could cope, so could I. My sister Rachael came from Brisbane for the weekend. She held my hand. I put on a brave face.

Matt Walker, my mate from skydiving school, came from the Gold Coast to support me. He made me laugh, arriving with a machine that filled the whole room with bubbles, much to the amusement of the medical team.

Ruth and Hamish called and shared my distress and frustration. They asked the questions I posed to myself every hour: 'Haven't you had enough by now, Josh? How do you keep going?' I wasn't too sure myself, though deep down I knew it was the love from my friends and family and those small, but yet perfect moments that life gives that held me together. I could talk honestly with them about my pain and sadness. My friends and family wanted me to enjoy my life, to run, laugh, have adventures and happiness and hang out with them. Every call from them was a joy, but so emotional too.

I spent 24 days in the Royal Melbourne Hospital, having multiple attacks, receiving morphine and fentanyl, breathing and meditating to calm my mind. Finally, the cardiologists found a blockage in my left main artery. It wasn't a significant one but it was causing the artery to spasm and restrict blood flow to the heart. The pain was so severe because this was a main artery feeding the heart and I was fortunate it hadn't closed right down because that would have killed off some of the heart muscle, with the risk of cardiac arrest. The treatments I'd received – chemo, radiation – and the GVHD had caused the damage to my arteries. Cancer treatment is so hard on the body and causes so much damage.

I was in a room with an Indian girl. She was 18 and having issues with her insurance company. Because she was a foreigner, the insurance company would not pay for her procedure, a cost of over $40,000. She cried at night because she had to find the money herself. I overheard her talking to the man who was supposed to be helping her with her insurance problems. It was tough to listen as this young sick woman struggled with this emotional and financial burden. The man seemed to be just ticking boxes on paper, saying repeatedly, 'This is all we can do.'

The next day I called the man into my room. I told him respectfully but firmly to do his job, make more calls and fight for this girl, because it was his job to help her. 'Stop telling her what the piece of paper says and look at her, human to human. Fight for her,' I said. 'She didn't ask to be here. You can do more.'

Two days later the insurance company agreed to pay for her procedure. I hope she's happy in life. Talking to her at night, hearing her laughter, kept me sane and helped me fight.

I don't care if I live or die: just make a decision.

The doctors had the longest patient meeting they'd ever had, discussing whether to put in a stent or perform heart bypass surgery on me. I had advanced disease in the left main artery and stenting that area was uncommon. I had written a note to my cardiologist, Will Williams. *Please just make a decision. I do not care if I live or die from what you do, as long as you can learn from me as a patient, and from the decision you make.*

After witnessing another attack, Dr Will Williams decided to take immediate action and put in the stent. The pain reduced dramatically, just like that. I was so relieved. Mum and Auntie Bernie were too. I'd spent nearly a month in the Royal Melbourne Cardiac Unit and of course my treatment at the Peter McCallum Centre had been put on hold. I'd lost a lot of weight. The GVHD had progressed and my skin was dry and tight and my muscles ached. I weighed 55 kg. I was back to square one. Again.

I was too weak to be on my own so my auntie's friends Tina and Rich took me in for six weeks while I continued my treatment. They became my Melbourne Mum and Dad, feeding me healthy food and caring for me. I gained some weight, got back on my feet, and my good humour returned, fuelled by Rich who was a very funny man. He could make a joke out of any situation and we got on great.

I wrote a thank-you message to Guy Lawrence who'd called the ambulance that morning at the Wim Hof Retreat and stayed with me until the medical team arrived. He sent me his podcast of the retreat. In the podcast, Guy was speaking to Dave O'Brien who owned a wellness centre in Melbourne called 5th Element Wellness. The centre had a scientific and holistic approach to wellness, was big on whole foods, gut health, the Wim Hof Method, cold and heat therapy, movement, strength training, meditation, natural supplementation and blood and stool analysis, all integrated under the same roof. I was excited, knowing this was the place I'd been looking for since my diagnosis six years earlier.

I heard the passion in Dave's voice when he spoke about health, saying there was no such thing as monotherapy. The way he spoke about holistic medicine, backing it up with scientific reasoning and evidence, ignited a spark for me. It was a calling.

I knew there was no one-hit answer to gaining back my health and wellness. I'd read and experienced enough to know that a number of elements working together cohesively was the key to restoring health and strength. As I listened to Dave, I felt he was reading my mind so I called and made an appointment to see him.

The 5th Element

I walked into 5th Element Wellness with a keen sense of curiosity. I prayed to God that this place would help me. My research and intuition had led me to these people, who knew the human body and could provide me with the nutrition and tools I needed to rebuild my immune system.

5th Element Wellness looked like an old workshop full of gym equipment, not at all what I'd expected. A big, strong man with a grey straggly beard come up and said, 'Josh, is that you?'

'Yeah, mate,' I said and he picked me up, hugged me and said,

'Mate, you're a fucking inspiration! I've been wondering how you were!'

Mark Kluwer was like a pirate who'd found his treasure. Despite his size, Mark, a gym member who'd also been at the Wim Hof retreat, was a gentle man who wore his heart on his sleeve and we became good friends. I was shown into an office where I met Dave O'Brien. I sat down and Dave began to share his extensive knowledge. He told me all about the gut, good and bad bacteria, and how our hormones have a huge impact on our body with different food we eat. We talked about everything 5th Element Wellness could offer and it was music to my ears. It all made sense. Deep down I knew this was the place to help me to heal and recover from all my treatments. Dave was an intelligent man, grounded and focused. He knew that hard work and dedication brought success.

Dave took my body measurements and set up a programme tailored to my requirements. The aim was to unravel my tight body and boost my immune system to its optimal level with real food, natural supplements and appropriate exercise. He became my mentor and I fed off every word he said. I trusted him completely.

The macro-nutrient plan was designed to help rebuild my immune system and body. Plenty of vegetables, good fats, slow cooked and offal meats were on the menu, with various supplements to reduce inflammation. Dave set me up with my trainer, Anthony Masino. Anthony's knowledge and passion for helping people overcome a life obstacle was inspiring and he gave me hope of regaining some quality of life. We became good friends, sharing thoughts about life and our interests. 5th Element became my new home. I wished I had found them earlier but thought, better late than never. I was determined to make the most of my experiences there.

Ice baths, bone broths, and lamb shanks for breakfast
Even though my body was still recovering from the heart attacks, Dr Simon Harrison, my doctor at Peter Mac, wanted to restart the

extracorporeal photopheresis treatment. The treatment was now out to three weekly and it was time to return to New Zealand. I was enjoying my time and newfound friends at 5th Element though I knew I would be back in three weeks' time. I planned to continue training in Greymouth at a local gym and catch up with Dave, Anthony and the team when I was in Melbourne.

After an arduous six months in Melbourne I had mixed emotions about leaving. I'd miss the comfort and reassurance provided by my new community at 5th Element. However, the excitement of going home increased as the day of departure drew near. I was looking forward to being back in the harmony of the West Coast nature, where my body and mind thrived, as well as sleeping in my own bed, being with my family and seeing my brother Jake.

Back home in Greymouth I caught up with my massage practitioner and good friend Dave Gordon. Dave is incredible at his job, with magic hands that helped ease the torment and unravel my tight and steely 'glued-up' body. I was on a mission to regain health, body and mind. I made bone broths, ate lamb shanks for breakfast and had four meals a day with good fatty meats and plenty of vegetables. I cut out all sugar, coffee, gluten, processed foods and hydrogenated vegetable oil. All pro-inflammatory foods. Every morning I got out of bed, straight into a three-minute cold shower followed by some Wim Hof breathing, then my stretching routine. Once a week I loaded up the bathtub with 50kg of ice and Hamish and I took a 5 to 10-minute ice bath.

I had a purpose and a routine. I was focused and determined like I was training for the Commonwealth Games again.

This time I was training for my life.

The baths and cold immersions were life-changing and worked wonders for my body. For two or three hours afterwards I felt good, alive, as if I'd never had cancer, ever. I was sprinting up and down my back lawn with Hamish, doing wolf howls, laughing like a kid with the strength of ten men.

The ice baths gave me a positive focus, a sense of elation, pushing, achieving. I dug deep, determined to do the best I could. They decreased the inflammation in my body, improved my immune system – especially the neutrophils, our main pathogen fighters – and increased the release of dopamine, a hormone that helps us feel good.

I was addicted. The nutritious food, the cold therapy, supplements, yoga, sauna and meditation were, collectively, restoring my crippled body. I had a long way to go but knew with the ECP treatment at Peter McCullum and the practices Dave instilled in me I was on the right path and had complete faith in Dave, Anthony and 5th Element Wellness.

Greymouth–Christchurch–Melbourne and back

The travel back and forth for treatment every month at Peter Mac was exhausting. My body was still not up to it, though I was slowly getting stronger, I did my best with the help of family and friends. I was blessed to have Mum and Dad taking care of me. Mum bought the food I needed, which took a considerable financial burden off me.

There was a routine for treatment week. First, I drove from Greymouth to Christchurch, stopping at Lake Pearson for a swim. I loved the feel of the cold water, being in nature, and couldn't help letting out some wolf howls. One time an astonished American tourist said, 'Hey man, are you okay?' and I replied, 'Yeah, bro, I just love being alive,' and started laughing aloud. The dude probably thought I was on drugs because he beat a hasty retreat.

I'd arrive at either my Auntie Rosie's house or my good friend Alex Mackenzie's in Christchurch where the lamb shanks were always ready for our dinner. Aunt Rosie had always been there for me. She'd seen my pain firsthand, knew instinctively what I needed, and was really happy to see me doing well.

Next morning, depending where I was staying, either Auntie Rosie or Alex would drive me to the airport at 4 am for the flight to Melbourne. It was often a kick in the teeth going through Customs as the photo ID scanner often did not recognise my face because the pigmentation had disappeared. It was always a reminder of how much I had changed physically. My good mate Paddy or his wife Frances would meet me and take me to my apartment at The Quest. By now I'd be exhausted and wanted to go to bed but I'd still need groceries so I'd walk weary and tired to the supermarket, passing by hundreds of people in a city that felt like a mosh pit, saying in my head, fuck off, fuck off, I hated being around so many people.

My exhaustion was profound. I'd be like a zombie on the sidewalk – eyes bloodshot, feeling like they were full of broken glass, mouth dry because I couldn't make saliva due to the radiation treatment and the GVHD, my body pleading with me to rest. I called the supermarket crazy mart because so many people crammed into the one shop. I'd purchase all I needed for the week, head back to the apartment, jump into the cold shower and straight to bed.

It was never easy to get the sleep I longed for. My head would pound like a jackhammer, eyes and mouth bone dry, and cramps would take about three hours to subside. I'd tussle with them until my body finally relented and I could drift off for a few hours.

Treatment would begin the next day. As I struggled awake, my mind would say, Get the fuck out of bed, man! But my body needed rest. It would take all of my energy and willpower to drag my fragile body to the shower.

The cold water would transform me and within minutes Josh was awake, smiling, hungry and wondering what all that fuss was about. The cold gave me the energy to start my day and head off for treatment.

The familiar place and the apheresis team always put a smile on my face. Two needles in each arm, blood drawn, separated, exposed to ultraviolet light and infused back into me.

Drained afterwards, I'd stagger back to the apartment, stretch, breathe and sleep.

The next day I'd rest, go to 5th Element and catch up with the team, assess my body, get a new programme from Dave, and exercise, meditate, talk and laugh with Anthony. The programme was bringing out the best in me. It wasn't always easy and sometimes I'd be crying in Dave's office, thinking I wasn't making any progress, but he assured me I was, telling me to stick with the protocol and compare myself to the Josh who first walked in the doors at 5th Element – not the Josh before cancer. His words went a long way to help me accept myself for who I was right now, and to see how far I'd really come. Soon I'd get the results I was after.

I always caught up with Mark Kluwer and his wife Julie during the week. They were like parents to me and Mark was the man who really inspired me to keep moving forward. He was passionate and enthusiastic about life. I respected and loved him.

Another day of treatment then back on the plane home, Auntie Rosie waiting to meet me in Christchurch as always. I'd stay the night and check in with my good friend Dr Peter the next day. Most of the time Peter and I just talked and caught up, nothing much about cancer or treatment, but more about my quality of life and what I was doing. On one my trips home from Melbourne I was in Peter's office discussing how treatment week went, soon the conversation shifted to talking about Napolean Bonapart for at least 30 minutes. That's how it was with Peter, I left laughing to myself and thinking how nice it was to not just talk about medical stuff. Dr Peter had been with me since Day One and I was grateful for the relationship I had with him.

On one occasion during treatment week I got talking to another patient, it's always great to meet new people and to share stories about their journeys. It gives me ideas about what they are doing for themselves outside of treatment. One man I met told me about what he was doing for his dry eyes, he obviously could see mine were extremely red and inflamed. He suggested I use 'autologus serum drops'* – made from my own blood – 'crazy', I thought. He said they had a positive effect on his eyes, reducing the dryness. When I got home I asked Dr Peter for a script for them.

Finally, the drive home to Greymouth. This was always the best part of treatment week. The drive itself was like a welcome home and lifted my spirits. New Zealand was paradise and I fell in love again every time I drove that road. I never got tired of it. Snow-capped mountains, fresh clean air. I forgot all about Melbourne, my treatment, my past. Filled with a deep appreciation for life and how far I'd come, I'd pull up at Lake Pearson and feel the cold, silky water enfold me. Time for wolf-howling with tears of gratitude on my cheeks. I wasn't jumping from a plane, or running 25 km on a hill. I wasn't on top of Mt Everest, but I was pain-free for that moment, alone, in a beautiful cold, clear lake. It was so simple, but to me it was perfect.

---

* Autologus serum drops are made from your own blood, the red blood cells and clotting factors are removed, leaving behind the diluted blood serum. The serum produces a tear substitute that contains many important growth factors and nutrients normally found in healthy tears. The 'blood drops' as I called them worked so well! They didn't fix my eyes but reduced the dryness, inflammation and redness by 30 to 40 per cent. I was so happy to have some relief.

PART FOUR
TODAY

The only thing that is
constant is change.

— HERACLITUS

Meeting Sibille

One treatment week the routine changed dramatically. On the flight to Melbourne I sat next to a pretty girl. The plane was full apart from one seat between us. I said to her, 'Hello, how was your day? She pulled her headphones out, surprised, and said, 'What?' I repeated my words and she laughed and said, 'Oh yes, it was fine.' I could tell by her accent she wasn't a New Zealander. Sibille was from Switzerland and travelling though Australia and New Zealand. She asked what I was doing in Melbourne. I told her I was visiting my brother who'd recently moved there. I didn't tell her the truth because I thought this woman I'd just met wouldn't want to hear my life story.

We kept talking and in the course of conversation she mentioned she was an oncology nurse who looks after cancer patients, so I told her why I was flying to Melbourne. She was intrigued by my treatment and I asked if she'd like to observe my session the following day. She agreed with such enthusiasm I knew that Sibille was special. I mean, how many women on holiday would want to see someone have their blood taken out and put back in?

Little did I know this would be our first date.

We hung out for the week, finding we had a lot in common. We had dinners together, enjoyed the city, and on my last day there, walked to Fitzroy Park and shared our last moments. We kissed and I couldn't believe this beautiful girl was attracted to me, given how I looked and especially after hearing about my life. I'd made up my mind it was rubbish, old news, and thought no one would want to be with me ever again.

Later on, Sibille came to Greymouth. We spent a week together and fell in love. I'd never expected to love again after Clara. Sibille is a beautiful, kind, funny woman who has such empathy for the people she meets in her everyday work.

Pure, unexpected moments, like meeting this woman on a plane ride to Melbourne, take away the pain I've suffered and reassure me how good life is. If you keep pushing through the pain, holding onto the love, soon something good will come. Sibille understands me; she knows my past without having been there. She has now received her New Zealand visa to come and live with me. We're madly in love.

November 2018

Today I still continue to receive treatment in Melbourne, flying back and forth. It's exhausting and there are days when I don't want to get on the plane and want to stop the treatment, but this is my life and I accept my life for what it is. The Graft Vs Host Disease in my body is stable, but I still get treatment, indefinitely for now.

As I sit here in Melbourne on a warm sunny afternoon, I look back on my past and towards the future. I conjure up those distant memories, when I lay curled in my hospital bed, crying in pain. I bring the past into this moment. It is an old friend who has taught me so much. At times, it was an enemy that I hated, but the pain I've endured has given me this time, right now, to be grateful and appreciate this moment.

I'm exhausted and hungry and yet I can sit with the warm air wrapped around my neck, the sun beating down on my face, and embrace it with a smile of complete appreciation because I know what it's like to have this taken away from me. A tear runs down my cheek as I realise how far I've come. Even though much was taken away, much was given.

I am alive, and have found freedom from within through the pain I've suffered, endured, spat and laughed at. Now I totally embrace the pain because this is life. I love this person, Josh Komen. I stood up when I was bashed down. I cried, vented my anger, screamed like a naked, lost child longing for his mother's hand. I'm content with the life I've had and continue to live.

How grateful I am to be me, in a position to suffer in comfort. I'm not in a war zone, not in a concentration camp! I have a warm bed, great friends, a beautiful girlfriend and a loving family. I can't complain, I have no right to. I have things in my life that many do not. My body may not function well, but I have love and support and that's what life is about.

There will be more hard days to come. For now, time is mine. I'll keep going because I love this life. I accept death for what it is, and when it comes calling, I'll greet it with a smile because I've given life my all.

I'm excited about my future with Sibille. She fills me with joy and will be here in time for Christmas. I feel as though I'm starting my life again, right now, with someone by my side to hold my hand, wipe my tears and get me back on my feet. Having someone in my corner, cheering me on, makes the journey less painful, the path easier, life far more peaceful. How good it is to be in love!

What keeps me moving forward? What lights the inner flame to carry on when it becomes so tough? It's the love, given so freely, by the incredible people I've met, from my early days as a no-worries young kid with bare feet and a shovel over my shoulder, all the way along this roller coaster ride called life. It's my mother's hand that held mine so tight, the unconditional love of my brother and sister, and my father's words, 'You're never alone, Josh.'

There have been many lonely times, but my family and friends were always with me in my heart and mind. If I closed my eyes, I could see their smiles or teary eyes, hear their laughter, and feel the deep love that brought me back from the brink of death and made me carry on when I wanted to give up. Pain taught me to share my deep, inner thoughts, and allow these people to pick me up.

Life is still far from easy, but it would be much harder without the blessings of love, the kind, caring people, and my hard-won life skills.

Sometimes I lost sight of this love. I had to search for its smallest fragments, gather them up, feel love grow again, vibrating through my body, over and over, like the beat of a loud drum.

I wear my heart on my sleeve these days and share my problems with family and friends. I trust, I cry, I'm no longer the hard man who can't vent his feelings. When my energy is low or my mood is off, I relax into various breathing exercises or jump into a cold river, lake or ice bath. When I'm lost or confused about my life I meditate and pray.

Life's small, perfect moments are profound and rewarding, like the soft breeze and sunshine on my face, a smile from a stranger, the song of birds in the distance, crying with love in a cold, clear lake, or a chance meeting with a girl on a plane. They fill my heart to the brim. I live for these unexpected moments. This is how I know life is good, and worth every twist, turn, and up and down I faced on the road to get here.

I embrace all that life has given me. I am healing, alive. I have love in my heart and the confidence to go forward. When you least expect it, if your heart and mind are open and willing, something good will fall into your lap.

Embrace these moments life gives us.

Love like your life
depends on it because
it does.

— ANITA MOORJANI

'Consider it pure joy, my brothers and sisters, whenever you face trials of many kinds because you know that the testing of your faith produces perseverance. Let perseverance finish its work so that you may be mature and complete, not lacking anything.'

JAMES 1:2–4

Acknowledgments

Writing this book has been no easy task. It meant I had to relive the memories, feel the pain, and cry all over again. I couldn't have got this far without my loving family who were always there, picking me up and supporting me in every respect along the way, and putting up with my shit! Mum, Dad, Rachael and Jacob, thank you for your unconditional love.

To my friends – you know who you are – thank you for your voices and presence that have helped me on this journey.

I couldn't have written this book without my new-found friend, editor and mentor, Jane Bissell, a lady who has also endured the cancer battle. Her patience and encouragement on those frustrating writing days helped me open my laptop and keep the writing flowing. Thank you so much for your kindness, your writing wisdom, and for helping me write this book. You're a Superstar, Jane!